PERCEPTUAL
HYPNOSIS

A Spiritual Journey Toward Expanding Awareness

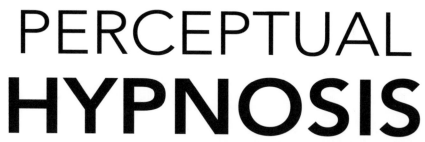

Fredrick Woodard, DCH,PhD

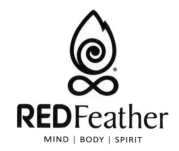

REDFeather

MIND | BODY | SPIRIT

Other Schiffer Books on Related Subjects:

UFO and Alien Management: A Guide to Discovering, Evaluating, and Directing Sightings, Abductions, and Contactee Experiences. Dinah Roseberry. ISBN: 978-0-7643-4606-4

Complete Meditation. Stephen Kravette. ISBN: 978-0-91491828-8

Very Practical Meditation. Serene West. ISBN: 978-0-89865006-8

Within the Power of Universal Mind. Rochelle Sparrow & Cortney Kane. ISBN: 978-0-7643-3786-4

Designed by Molly Shields
Cover design by Brenda McCallum

Type set in Avenir LT Std (TT)/Times New Roman

ISBN: 978-0-7643-5310-9
Printed in China

Published by Red Feather Mind Body Spirit
An Imprint of Schiffer Publishing, Ltd.
4880 Lower Valley Road
Atglen, PA 19310
Phone: (610) 593-1777; Fax: (610) 593-2002
E-mail: Info@schifferbooks.com
Web: www.schifferbooks.com

For our complete selection of fine books on this and related subjects, please visit our website at www.schifferbooks.com. You may also write for a free catalog.

Schiffer Publishing's titles are available at special discounts for bulk purchases for sales promotions or premiums. Special editions, including personalized covers, corporate imprints, and excerpts, can be created in large quantities for special needs. For more information, contact the publisher.

We are always looking for people to write books on new and related subjects. If you have an idea for a book, please contact us at proposals@schifferbooks.com.

DEDICATION

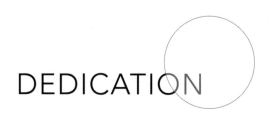

This book is a labor of love dedicated to those individuals who have shared their problems, suffering, and knowledge with me. They have given me spiritual gifts that I will always cherish. Many wonderful people have inspired me to write about this topic—far too many to list here. I want to thank all of them. I especially want to thank a few individuals who have had a great impact on my spiritual journey and on the psychological development of my soul's evolution: My maternal grandfather, William Abel, for encouraging me to never give up! My mother and father for their sacrifices in raising me and enabling me to achieve what I have so far. Victoria for coming along and awakening my greater potential. Georgiana for reminding me about my potential. Father Edmund O'Brien for mentoring me with his spiritual support throughout the years. My Uncle Frederick Woodard for giving his life for our country. Dr. Anne Cohen Richards for her support in encouraging me to put my ideas into manuscripts for journal articles and books. Dr. David Underwood, Dr. Paul Cunningham, Dr. Pierre Dionne, Dr. Donna Hastings, and Dr. Robert Kaladish for their support and encouragement. My Aunt Beverly Strong for being there for me. My many cousins, the Kirks, the Lefebvre families, and the Woodard families, for their emotional support through the years. Charles and Tim Shay, my distant cousins and descendants of Chief Madockawando, for sharing their spiritual experiences with me.

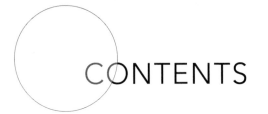

CONTENTS

Amnesia, Hypermnesia, Paramnesia, and Crytomnesia
Positive Hallucinations
Negative Hallucinations
Analgesia and Anesthesia
Post-hypnotic Suggestion
Catalepsy
Subconscious Manifestations
Somnambulism

ACKNOWLEDGMENTS

Dr. Errol Leifer and Dr. Shelley Stokes for allowing me in my doctorate at CSPP in Fresno, California, to work freely on new ideas I had formulated about hypnosis and perception. Drs. Carol and Douglas Ammons of Ammon Scientific for working with me on numerous journal articles that are fundamental to my writing and research. Dr. Thomas Gooding and Ellen Winkler for reading my manuscript and providing succinct commentary. Dinah Roseberry and Peter Schiffer for their expertise in publishing this work. Dr. Anne Cohen Richards for her support of my writing and her editorial suggestions. Carol Haywood for typing the original footnotes in the first draft of the manuscript. Gregor Bernard for his illustrations that materialized my experiences. Murray Hensch for the photograph of the author. Kari Voight for editing the manuscript. And most of all, I acknowledge the pioneers of the study of human experience who allowed me the freedom to write this book by paving the path ahead of me. To all the remarkable souls who have laid these foundations for a greater understanding of our psychological depth: Milton Erickson, William James, Carl Jung, Fredrich Mesmer, Wilhelm Reich, and others of kindred spirit who have fought for freedom of thought and expression of the truth, despite attacks based on popular opinion or consensus thinking that have dismissed, quieted, or even threatened them in their quest to know more and share their insights.

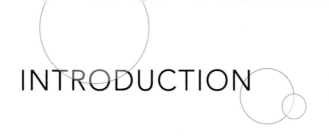

INTRODUCTION

As the wise Solomon saith, Wisdom entereth not into the malicious mind,
and that knowledge without conscience is but ruin of the soul.[1]

—Francois Rabelais

This book takes you on a journey of discovery about a subject not well
understood by people in our culture or even by the majority of professionals in
the field of psychology—that is, hypnosis and its relationship to spirituality. My
hope is that as you read this book you will learn about the perceptual process of
hypnosis, understand what it is and what it isn't, how this framework can be used
with a spiritual intention, and how it can potentially change your life.

In seeking fulfillment in your life, perhaps you have asked yourself questions
such as these:

- Am I using my full potential?
- Is there something deeper and more meaningful to life that I am missing?
- Are there different realities that I cannot see?
- Can I overcome the limitations in my life?
- Can I find ways to change my destiny?
- Am I in control of my own mind?

If you have pondered any of these or similar questions, you have already begun
exploring your human and spiritual potential, and this book might provide some
answers and open a simpler and more efficient path through a personal growth
process as you read through these pages.

As the beginning of the twentieth century saw the joining of science and hypnosis,
the twenty-first century has seen a unity of hypnosis and spirituality in a way that
has not occurred for centuries—not since the work of Franz Mesmer in the 1700s
and his predecessor Paracelsus, a German-Swiss Renaissance physician, botanist,
and alchemist in the early 1500s. In other words, we are only rediscovering what
we already have known and forgotten. Some of the spiritual exercises in Paracelsus's
ancient writings are currently labeled "cognitive behavioral" techniques and are
now seen as science, but stripped of their original spirituality. While spirituality was
being ignored, the great minds of President Abraham Lincoln, authors Mark Twain
and William Blake, Dr. William James (an American psychologist and father of
American psychology), and Dr. Wilhelm Wundt (a German psychologist who created
the first psychology laboratory), among others, explored and advanced the understanding
and knowledge of various spiritual phenomena such as telepathy, spirits, and

clairvoyance. Since these experiences are not measurable, many scientists—that is those still espousing the mechanistic model of reality—insist that they don't exist. Though paranormal experiences and hypnosis resist some types of examination, they are both examples of everyday phenomena and aspects of the Universe that we all have the potential to access and use to enhance life.[2] They are certainly legitimate subjects for scientific exploration.

I first was exposed to hypnosis while exploring spiritual experiences in my twenties. Hypnosis was a way of re-entering this peaceful and creative space within myself. I was hypnotized by four important people in my life that I respected:

- A shamanic healer
- A certified hypnotist
- A Washington, DC, homicide investigator
- A professor of psychology who was also a clinical psychologist

I began to practice self-hypnosis to further develop my spiritual awareness. It was a way of encouraging my inner self to connect with the outside world in a more "active" rather than reactive way. By active I mean I learned to pause and to discern what was really happening rather than just responding unconsciously or mindlessly to people and situations. I began to learn to take control of my mind and my being in a new and more rewarding way, no longer the victim of outside influences that were not meaningful to me. I began to learn that I could control my thoughts and reactions rather than being controlled by them. I was expanding myself, healing, feeling empowered. And I came to realize that this hypnosis I had been exposed to had not only increased my spiritual awareness but also had much potential for healing the world.

I first learned the seed to this powerful healing ability in a simple test: seeing if I was able to be hypnotized by Dr. Al Krasner, author of *The Wizard Within* and founding father of the American Institute of Hypnotherapy. There were two possible reactions that could have occurred when I was asked to clasp my hands tightly closed and then to try to release them during hypnosis. One reaction was that I might perceive myself as able to open my hands and thus fail to accomplish this hypnotic task and prevent the perceived control from someone else, which, by the way, is exactly what I did. I thought this meant that I had failed to experience hypnosis and had triumphantly defeated the hypnotist's request. However, I came to realize through Dr. Krasner's excellent training that, in hypnosis, I was really in control—not the hypnotist. I realized that I was unable to unclasp my hands when I listened and followed the instructions correctly, i.e., my hands would only move and open when I was thinking they could, and when I was thinking they could not open, then they could not open. I had to imagine or think something was possible before I was able to create or act on it. No magic was involved. For every individual, perceptual awareness harnesses this great personal and creative power.

With such new knowledge in my awareness, I began to explore the academic theories of hypnosis and spirituality and read a considerable amount of the scientific literature on these topics. Yet there always seemed to be something missing in the explanations, something that just didn't fit for me. Then I came upon the work of Drs. Donald Snygg and Arthur Combs and their perceptual psychology. Perceptual psychology originated in the 1940s and continues in educational psychology in the present through such educators as Dr. Anne Cohen Richards and Dr. Mark Wasicsko. This form of psychology understood persons and their behavior through the lens of perceptual awareness. Humans were seen as having a paramount need to be as adequate as possible in their lives, based on their perceptions and personal meanings. (I will expound further on this theory in the chapters ahead.) I realized that most approaches to hypnotism seemed to be more interested in external control and manipulation rather than emphasizing and understanding internal influences occurring within the subject. There seemed to be a truth about this inner way of understanding hypnosis and spirituality that I found self-evident and not contrary to my intuition of what I personally experienced and discovered.

I then developed a new approach to understanding the hypnotic process of expanding perceptual awareness—termed *perceptual hypnosis*—the gist of which I defined in a series of journal articles.[3] I formed the foundation of my understanding of hypnosis through my own encounters with altered states and spiritual exercises. Specifically, I experienced being hypnotized and received training by lay hypnotists and psychologists. I have utilized hypnosis with clients as a lay hypnotist and as a psychologist, and have conducted research on hypnosis with many volunteers. I have also experienced altered states through Eastern meditation; Native American ceremonies on Indian Island in Old Towne, Maine; and at a sweat lodge at Tule River reservation in Porterville, California. I have attended psychic development classes throughout the country and have witnessed numerous esoteric activities with various groups. All of these spiritual experiences helped me obtain an understanding of how our perceptual awareness develops and opens us to more accurate perceptions of our Universe. As a responsible person, I did not speak about something I had not personally experienced or researched. I collected information on these particular subjects, such as hypnosis and spirituality, while exploring critical evaluations of the subject matter. I also sought to experience these phenomena in everyday life for myself. I could not deny the genuineness of my spiritual experiences, so I sought to investigate, research, and understand them. In seeking the truth about life (accurately perceiving), we can all find truth while taking different paths, expanding beyond the immediate physical environment.

These spiritual experiences seemed to bring the past and the future into a new perspective for me. So many invisible influences that have led to this very moment we are experiencing now. The past held many unknown and forgotten secrets, and the future had greater potential than I had previously thought. The work of Carl Jung claims that we carry our ancestors' histories and knowledge in our physical bodies, if not our souls. I often wondered how many of my ancestors or my readers' ancestors gave their very lives so we could be here today. When I mentioned this idea to a number of my clients, quite a few of them responded positively and with a renewed faith in their own lives. We often forget who we really are!

Others discuss the possibilities of past lives and future lives and experiences from many different dimensions. These aspects of the Universe open up diverse possibilities, while other forces seek to keep us trapped, focusing only on our physical reality and its many created limitations.

When I was investigating my family genealogy, a very exhaustive endeavor in both time and labor, I was surprised at the many false family histories, recording errors, and outright misinformation published in printed books and later on Internet sites, which were accepted as true by those seeking quick and easy solutions to difficult problems.[4, 5] Too many people were willing to invest neither their own time nor their own money for something they genuinely desired to know, or they were unaware that they were not seeking the original sources. The truth is out there, but it is not always a simple process. Meanwhile, others haphazardly put names together that don't go together.

It is also synchronistic that I found, while researching my lineage, that I was descended from a very ancient spiritual line—great-grandson to shaman and Grand Chief Madockawando of the Abenaki Nation, the Merovingian Kings, Charlemagne, and the House of Judah. No wonder spirituality and freedom of thought has always been a major theme in my life!

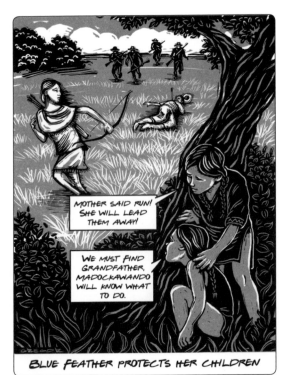

MOTHER SAID RUN!
SHE WILL LEAD
THEM AWAY!

WE MUST FIND
GRANDFATHER,
MADOCKAWANDO
WILL KNOW WHAT
TO DO.

BLUE FEATHER PROTECTS HER CHILDREN

In Chapter 8, I tell the story of a clinical psychologist who was asked to create a bogus diagnosis for a Native American girl and who subsequently reported this incident to the state's mental health board, resulting in the clinical director's dismissal. The girl was the daughter of a chief at a local reservation and her father was being pressured to release land to the local government. This psychologist's heroic

*Blue feather protects
her children.*

behavior affected me deeply as I was joining the ranks of professionally trained psychologists, expected to help people. It also made a powerful impression on me as a great-grandson of Chief Madockawando, Grand Sachem of the Abenaki Nation in the 1690s in Maine.[6] This genetic link led me to feel connected to the injustice being perpetrated against the Native American girl. I felt evermore committed to the principle that the focus of my work was to empower individuals as a way of enhancing a diverse and supportive community through more accurately perceiving our place in the Universe.

One reason for writing this book was to dispel misunderstandings about hypnosis. One of my clients voiced a fear that he would "slip away and not come back" if he allowed himself to be hypnotized. Expressions such as "let him put me under" or "while I was under hypnosis" imply that some magical force is employed to keep a person in an altered level of awareness during hypnosis. But in reality you achieve greater awareness and gain more control over your mind and life—not less control— during the hypnotic experience. Thus, you become dehypnotized from many external influences that have shaped your views since birth.

Despite its long history, hypnotic therapy has eluded understanding by the average person. For example, recently a middle school client usually accompanied by his mother to a psychotherapy session was brought to his appointment by his aunt. She positioned herself in the lobby so that I was unable to see her. Her nephew explained that she knew I was a hypnotist, and she didn't want to look into my eyes because she was afraid I would hypnotize her. Introducing people to hypnosis or expanding their awareness is not that easy, however. One reason that most people have failed to grasp what hypnosis is all about is that they have been trying to tackle the experience through cognitive analysis, rather than approaching it as a holistic experience. This book endeavors to present both an intellectual and experiential encounter in a holistic framework.

As you gain new understanding of your hypnotic abilities, it is possible to embrace your unique individuality while still being universally conscious and sensitive at the same time. In this way, you magnify both a greater individuality and an empathy for others. With such an expanded perceptual awareness, you can avoid the philosophical traps of being too all-inclusive (at the cost of individuality) or too individualistic (ignoring human commonalities). While there are many external influences that lead one to a fear of being different, we are all unique, just like a snowflake or a fingerprint. Some people gravitate toward the familiar and attack that which is different or try to force conformity on those unique souls, thus maintaining rather than enhancing the self through fear.

Educating people about hypnosis has been bungled by some professionals much the way that Buscaglia's (1972) "Animal School" analogy shows general education being bungled by a school board. Buscaglia's story is about a school board-mandated curriculum that teaches the same skills to all animals, but fails to be effective because, for instance, a giraffe isn't designed to swim in a pond like a frog and a frog isn't designed to eat leaves off the high branches of trees, the way a giraffe is.[7]

Buscaglia's story illustrates how forcing specific standards that work for some onto others is not always scientifically sound and is rather rigid. Most people can be hypnotized, since all hypnosis is really fundamentally self-hypnosis. However, if someone doesn't want to experience hypnosis, then hypnosis will not occur. Perceptual awareness shows us how there are many ways of seeing and dealing with events in different contexts. We must remain flexible and multidimensional in our perceptions, or we will become estranged from the full benefits of our experiences. In fact, rigidity and single-dimensionality will lead us to devolve rather than evolve. The most effective aspect of hypnosis is a perceptual process rich in imagination and creativity rather than the stifling hive mentality.

Unfortunately, you might still be afraid of hypnosis because you do not understand it. You might fill in the gaps of your knowledge with many false beliefs because of your own fear or suggestions by others. What is a suggestion? It is verbal encouragement to alter your perceptual awareness and change what you are discerning in the Universe. You might be afraid of losing control, become unconscious, and do something contrary to your normal waking conduct, such as revealing secrets to others. The sad consequence of falling prey to unfounded fears based on myths about hypnosis is that it leads you to avoid a powerful tool available to enhance your life.

An important point in our discussion of spiritual hypnosis is the concept of perceptual awareness. Perceptual awareness can be defined as your capacity to understand and interpret your personal world through differentiation—by differentiation, I mean identifying an aspect of your Universe. It's the innate ability you possess to apprehend your personal world and the Universe through the powers of your perception—to become aware.

So how does changing your perceptual awareness during hypnosis affect your exercise of free will? During the unfolding of the hypnotic process, you are giving full attention to your internal world. You will not do anything against your personal beliefs and values, since you perceive them to be true. You never lose control over your mind or actions as a result of such intensely focused perceptual awareness. Again, you become aware of how the outside influences and past experiences have affected your free will, thus expanding your freedom of thought and action in this moment.

Your self-image can improve through using perceptual hypnosis. It brings forth self-control over how and what you perceive in the Universe. It allows you to see yourself differently, thus bringing positive change, such as diminished fear when setting out to accomplish things. Becoming aware of more of your diverse perceptual possibilities may enable you to better understand what you still need to work on in terms of your personal growth. Understanding how perceptual awareness and hypnotic principles work together allows you to step back and see who you really are and what has been affecting your self-image as well as your self.

Perceptual hypnosis can help you to change a negative self-definition through raising your awareness of the ways that you create your own restrictions and traps. For example, those who use others to attain their goals are often afraid to reach a high level of success in their own lives because they fear others will ask for similar assistance from them. Other examples can include not taking risks in social situations to get to know new people, not going back to school because you're "too old," and being prejudiced against a different racial group. You are often blind to the perceptual fact that it is your own differentiations of your perceived Universe, either at higher levels of awareness or lower levels, that block out pieces of the Universe and allow you to perceive only limited aspects of it.

Perceptual hypnosis helps you investigate seemingly divergent aspects of the Universe and actually find the relationships that exist in them. It may be seen as similar to the work of a police detective attempting to reconstruct a crime as it happened at a given moment in time, allowing everyone involved to clearly and accurately discern what had taken place. Both are processes of seeking to accurately perceive the truth about aspects of the Universe and remove the illusions.

Perceptual hypnosis allows you to experience aspects of another's reality by enabling you to cross boundaries of consciousness you might have thought were fixed, or by joining in a shared point of view beyond the limits of your ego. It can help you understand how another person perceives you, and why others behave toward you as they do. Seeing something, or yourself, from different perspectives can go a long way toward increasing understanding between individuals, groups, cultures, and nations.

Exploring your own inner experiences can help you to bring more empathy and comprehension to your relationships. For example, as I see it, a diagnosis of mental illness can be influenced by an excessively negative perceived perspective or complete lack of knowledge about spiritual experiences. Let's look at the cases of two individuals who appear to experience the same phenomenon in very different contexts.

> **Case 1:** A male client at work watches his boss walk away from a conversation with a female co-worker. The man observes as the boss stops, then walks back and asks if this woman had called his name. She said, "Yes." She then continues her conversation with her boss. When that conversation has ended and the boss has walked away, my male client asked his coworker, "You didn't call his name, did you?" This woman stated: "No, but I thought it." The woman, considered psychic, communicated without actually calling out the boss's name, so that the boss "heard" her thoughts.

> **Case 2:** A female diagnosed as schizophrenic is in a basement of a group home doing her laundry. She comes upstairs and asks if the group home manager (the author) had called her name. The manager didn't call her name out loud but rather thought it in his mind.

The woman in Case 1 is considered spiritually gifted or psychic by some people. The woman in Case 2, labeled schizophrenic, is considered mentally ill by most. These both appear to be genuine examples of psychic experiences that some would classify as schizophrenic in nature. The "psychic" woman (Case 1) might seek out spiritual guidance or a mentor who has had similar experiences, while the "schizophrenic" woman (Case 2) will no doubt be treated by mental health professionals using medical and psychological interventions and explanations. Interestingly enough, research in cross-cultural studies demonstrate that other countries have a better success rate with treating schizophrenia than the United States. One possible reason for this difference could be that there is more acceptance of paranormal and spiritual experiences in those cultures. In addition, those cultures have more focus on internal experiences and have diverse meanings for spiritual, mental, and emotional suffering.

Many of the quotations in this book are from philosophers, psychologists, and researchers who lived at much earlier times in history. These passages might contain language considered sexist by today's standards, because the writers used male pronouns to refer to mankind at large or to both genders. The original language of the quotations has been retained, but does not represent any gender bias on the part of the author or publisher of this book. We have both made an effort to ensure the book uses gender-neutral pronouns, gives illustrative examples that include cases featuring both females and males, and avoids sexual stereotyping of roles.

Now, let's begin the journey into the world of hypnosis and spirituality. Remember, the process of understanding must include experience. The exercises that I've developed at the end of the chapters will take your reading to a deeper level. We will start with a simple relaxation and protection exercise to help you find that place within where hypnosis occurs. This is a standard exercise the reader should start before each subsequent exercise.

Through the use of such exercises, you may become more familiar with what hypnosis is and how one experiences self-hypnosis and meditation in everyday life. These simple exercises have lasting effects of improving health, removing stress, and allowing one to quiet her mind. The daily practice of hypnosis allows a person to increase an openness to learning, to become less reactive, and to obtain a more natural way of being closer to nature in awareness. This will be further enhanced by working with a hypnotherapist or a psychotherapist who uses hypnosis as a counseling tool.

SELF-HYPNOSIS EXERCISE

First, take a deep breath. Breathe deeply, slowly, and completely, taking in as much oxygen as you can. Count one, two, and three as you inhale or whatever number is comfortable for you to breathe as deeply, slowly, and as fully as you can. Next, hold your breath to a count of three or the number that is comfortable for you as you pause between inhalation and exhalation for the same number. Then, gently and slowly exhale completely to a count of three or the number that best suits your breathing. Over time you may expand this to a count of four or five while breathing and pausing. Do this breathing exercise a few times, relaxing as much as possible. Breathe fully so you let all the air in your lungs in and out each time you inhale and exhale. Relax into this rhythm and let your breathing become natural.

Focus on a deep bright purple, with fluorescent sparks of violet. Imagine this color (or another color you prefer with this same mixture of one shade deep and bright and another shade fluorescent) giving an effect of lightning bugs at night or glow-in-the-dark sparkling lights. Imagine as you close your eyes that these bright and fluorescent colors are moving slowly through your body as a fluid or as energy moving from your toes to the top of your head, swirling and massaging your being from the surface of your skin deep into your muscles and your bones and deeper into your inner self. Go slowly and allow each area of your body to relax and receive this light.

Say in your mind, as you imagine this color purple moving up from the soles of your feet to your toes, "My soles and toes are so relaxed." See this energy soaking through and penetrating deeply into your body and being as a light illuminates a room or as a sponge absorbs water. A dry sponge is stiff and inflexible, but once filled with water, it expands and becomes soft and flexible. Imagine any tension in your muscles released.

Picture any negative energy as black specks and gray smoke that travels up through your body and exits through an opening on top of your head into a ball. Notice your body and pay special attention to this mansion of your soul. Notice your breathing, notice your heartbeat, notice the different sensations and experience your body fully. Feel yourself relaxing more and more as the light you imagine moves up to the top of your foot and your ankles. Let the fluorescent sparks of violet light go wherever you feel tension, pain, irritation, or problems, allowing soothing, relaxing protection and healing into those areas. For example, if you have a broken bone or have a bruised or sore muscle, imagine these fluorescent sparks attracted to the spot that needs healing, just as moths are attracted to a street light. The fluorescent sparkles are soothing and enhancing to your body's ability to heal itself. Imagine this for a few moments.

Then imagine this colorful energy moving up to your lower legs, knees, and thighs. See this energy moving through your genitals, your buttocks, your abdomen, stomach, and your lower back. Feel how relaxing and soothing this colorful energy is to your treasured body. You are the protector and keeper of your body. You bring only nourishment and health to your body. Then move this energy up your fingers, palms, and back of your hands, your wrists, your lower arms, elbows, your upper arms, and up to your back and through your shoulders, merging to your neck. Go up through your stomach, chest and your back, and to your neck. Let your whole upper body relax. Imagine the muscles in your upper body relaxed. The energy moves deeper to the bones. Your organs are relaxed and soothed and cleansed with this energy.

Now your heart pumps perfectly, not too fast and not too slow—just right. Your emotions relax. Imagine all your neck muscles relaxing. Your jaw, face, and scalp and all the tiny muscles in your head relax. As this colorful light is moving up each part of your body, see any tension and stress as gray smoke or black specks or blobs leaving through the top of your head and forming a ball over your head. As you finish this relaxation, send this ball up into the sky and watch as it travels higher and higher. Just before it is out of sight, it disintegrates and vanishes into nothingness, where it can no longer do you or anyone else any harm. Say to yourself, "And harm to no one."

Then see a ball of white light coming from the heavens and hovering over your head. Allow that ball of light to glow and grow. See it descend upon you and completely envelop your whole body. Feel this light enter your body, this luminosity merge with you, and allow yourself to think of nothing else but this ball of light, feeling completely peaceful, tranquil, and calm. You are completely protected and relaxed.

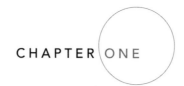

CHAPTER ONE

HOW YOU DEVELOP YOUR PERCEPTUAL AWARENESS

Since hate is with us still, I wish men love;
I wish, since hovering hawks still strive to kill,
The coming of the Dove.
And since the ghouls of terror and despair
are still abroad,
I wish the world once more within the care of
Those who have seen God.[8]

—Dr. Christopher Woodard

We begin with a look at the nature of individual consciousness. How are our perceptions and personal meanings formed? How do we organize our thoughts and relate to our world? How do we develop a personality? From the day we are born—some might say before then—we start to form our perceptions and meanings of the world or what I refer to as the "Universe," which I define as all the internal and external things and experiences that affect us that are both visible and invisible—invisible in that they transcend the physical earth. I choose the word "Universe" to describe what surrounds us, influences us, and interacts with us, since it is much more than just our physical environment and that should be recognized.

YOUR PERSONAL WORLD

Your parents were your first hypnotists. You were also hypnotized by the world you encountered, well before you realized it was happening. Your parents and other significant people helped you associate personal meanings and perceptions with your early experiences. Some of your current points of view you might have learned in an almost unconscious way: Crying will elicit a response. Big sisters don't like to share. Cats like to be petted; dogs don't like their tails pulled. And as you grew, the lessons became more complex; perhaps: Don't expect to be rich when you grow up. You must be married by a certain age. Men cannot cry. Or more positive messages may have come your way: You can do anything you put your mind to. People are essentially good. Develop your talents.

Most parents try to present the Universe as accurately as possible. As children, you either accepted or rejected their suggestions, and then you went about unconsciously or mindlessly replicating your early experiences as if you had special lenses to see through and observe the Universe. You noticed some things, were unaware of others, responding selectively to your world without consciously realizing you were doing so. Your parents' messages were your first posthypnotic suggestions. These posthypnotic suggestions were messages you seemingly learned from others, and you acted upon this knowledge later, often without being aware that you were given such suggestions. Family therapists refer to this process of parents shaping their children's perceptual awareness as "transgenerational patterns," first identified by Milton Erickson, a famous physician and hypnotist.

Even during simple conversation, suggestions may be given and accepted perceptually between two individuals. Did you ever notice that when one person begins to yawn, soon others around him or her also yawn? Hypnosis works through body messages as well as language—for instance, facial expressions, gestures, postures, movements, and aspects of the human voice. In addition, my research has found that bodily experiences during hypnosis are often exchanged in such a manner that you cannot describe or explain them.[9] David Harvey, author of *The Power to Heal*, provides a relevant example while discussing faith healing:

> In one [drug] trial in the United States of America, women complaining of sickness were given a potion that, by rights should have actually made them feel more nauseous [*sic*]. Through the magic of suggestion and expectation—they were told that the drug was an effective antidote to sickness—and the opposite occurred; they reported a cessation of nausea and said they felt much better.[10]

The "suggestion" in this case had a hypnotic effect. You might say that these experimenters were able to convey their suggestion on multiple levels of awareness to be effective. These other levels of your awareness operate automatically when the ego is either preoccupied or refusing to participate.

To demonstrate the various points of developing perceptual awareness and spiritual experience, I ask you to consider the movie *The Lion King* as an analogy. This is a movie where the main character is Simba, the son of Mufasa, king of the lions, and his mate, Sarabi. It focuses on a great analogy of becoming aware of the Universe with all its aspects, both good and bad, and learning how to overcome the many false obstacles placed in his way. From the time he was born, Simba began to explore and become curious about how the Universe works, and so he started in this way to develop his perceptual awareness. He learned cause and effect, boundaries, and labels for things. His guardians taught him well and provided him with protection from harm and helped him to understand his world. Simba began to differentiate and created a personal world I call the "perceived Universe," which consists of some of the actual aspects of the Universe along with distortions created by the cub and others in his life. His Uncle Scar made him falsely believe he was responsible for his father's death: He went with his uncle Scar for a surprise and was left in a canyon. Scar had Simba wait in the canyon for him. Meanwhile, Scar sent for the hyenas to start a stampede that would trap Simba and his father, Mufasa, in that canyon, from which they had no way to escape. Mufasa attempted to save his son by jumping and crawling up the walls of the cliff. He succeeded in getting his son to safety but fell back into the stampede himself. He made one more majestic attempt and began to crawl up the cliff walls but was killed by his own brother, Scar, who pushed him off the cliff. Not seeing how his father Mufasa had fallen to his death, Simba was told by Scar that it was he himself who was at fault for putting his father in danger. Then Scar sent the hyenas to kill Simba, but Simba escaped into the desert, where he remained for several years. Truthfully, Simba's behavior was influenced by this distorted perception of reality given to him by his uncle while he was exiled in the wilderness. Simba had to see through the illusions placed in his way and his own inner fears to defend his pride from destruction.

Drs. Donald Snygg and Arthur Combs, both psychologists who developed the phenomenal field theory in the 1940s, define what I call the perceived Universe as the phenomenal field. As they defined it:

> It is simply the Universe of naïve experience in which each individual lives, the everyday situation of self and surroundings which each person takes to be reality. To each of us the phenomenal field of another person contains much error and illusion and seems an interpretation of reality rather than reality itself; but to the individual himself his phenomenal field is reality, the only reality he can know.[11]

This perceptual theory and hypnosis explained throughout this book helps explain how Simba and you (the reader) have developed false and distorted perceptions that restrict and limit your potentials, but it is possible to develop strategies to see more clearly.

DIFFERENTIATION, NOT DISSOCIATION

You cannot focus on all aspects of your personal world at once. Differentiation is a process of magnifying aspects of your own perceived Universe (real and imagined) and the entire Universe (real). Drs. Snygg and Combs described it as ". . . a continual change in the perceptual field by the constant rise of new characters into figure and the constant lapse of others into ground. This process . . . is one of increased awareness of details and is, therefore, called differentiation."[12] Snygg went on to state that differentiation was the only human process occurring in the Universe.[13] And I believe it is the key to a greater understanding of hypnosis.

The Universe is evident in both your conscious awareness (called *figure*) and in low levels of your "unconscious" awareness (called *ground*). Ground is the background of your perceived Universe that you are typically unaware of at a specific moment, whether or not you can be aware intellectually that these aspects exert an influence on you. You cannot consciously perceive what is in ground. Figure is the aspect of experience you see or observe in your perceived Universe at any particular moment in time. Figure is like the fin of a shark or the tip of an iceberg, suggesting more but not revealing it. As an example, a soldier is taught how to fight consciously, but his intuition is that which helps him make better choices when he is consciously limited in awareness. This happens when he chooses between two cliffs to climb and picks the one that is safe, rather than the cliff guarded by heavily armed enemy soldiers, without consciously knowing the soldiers were there.

For example, if you place a number of items on the kitchen table and consider this table a perceived Universe or personal world, then a number of reactions may be triggered by these items. If you concentrate on just a single object—say your French press coffeemaker—and focus all of your attention on this object, it's possible to forget about the rest of the table to such an extent that the garlic press, ice cream scoop, and gravy boat will fade into the background. You may no longer be aware that these objects are even there. The object focused on is what is salient or "in figure" in your perceived Universe. You choose what you wish to see, differentiating what you see in just this manner, every day of your life.

The question becomes, how does your perceptual awareness work in your personal world and the Universe? You experience the Universe through differentiation. To better understand differentiation, consider that not all aspects of your perceived Universe are equally distinct. Your perceived Universe can include others—even others not in your physical environment, such as your deceased grandfather or a friend who moved away—as well as past events and your concepts of the future.

The process of differentiating creates varied levels of awareness. Using the kitchen table example, you may discard an object from the table and replace it with another, thus reorganizing your perceived Universe as the new object takes precedence over the other object (although the original object remains in the greater Universe). Your perceived Universe is constantly changing through differentiation, as aspects move from higher levels of awareness into lower levels and vice versa. Some aspects remain in higher levels of awareness for long periods of time, and others almost permanently remain in lower levels.

DIFFERENTIATION AND ITS AFFECTS

You can choose what you see. Your personal history and current need to maximize potential may allow you to see what always was present yet until now remained unobserved. You could be in the same place all of your life and suddenly see things for the first time, things that have always been there. For example, an owl might have frequently been perched in a tree in your front yard, yet not until you develop an interest in nature do you notice that owl. The owl remained out of conscious awareness in your perceived Universe, while other aspects were more interesting and dominated consciousness at higher levels of awareness. This may also be true for subjective experience, such as that related to spiritual phenomena.

Hypnosis can assist in reorganizing your perceived Universe, shifting what is in higher levels of conscious awareness and allowing you to perceive aspects of the Universe that have been at lower levels of awareness—to change your focus so that you become aware of the owl, or tune in to emotions you have been ignoring, or increase your awareness of relationship issues you have refrained from facing.

A client of mine, for example, drove to my office one day observing on his way to his appointment all the things that were yellow. He observed thirty-eight different objects that he had never noticed before, and it changed his perceptual awareness. Often you become too habitual in differentiating what is happening around you. Your awareness dulls. For example, after a serious car accident left a client in a cast for months and dependent on crutches, he began to observe many people using canes, crutches, and wheelchairs both on television and in his community. Sadly, he rarely ever noticed people in such circumstances prior to his accident. This happened to my editor, Dinah, when she began to have "fragrance sensitivity." Smells would send her into a cluster headache. She never knew how many people wore perfume (really strong) or how many candle isles there really were in every single store she went into! Smells that triggered her were *everywhere*!

Your ability to differentiate these levels of awareness may expand the scope of your mind so that you can, for example, recall memories you've forgotten or have more control over your emotions. The flexibility and shifting of your perceived Universe and self, along with altering levels of awareness through differentiation, may explain several phenomena:

- The altered state of the mind in meditation
- Sleepwalking disorder
- Paranormal phenomena
- The hypnotic state
- Lucid dreaming (being aware that you are dreaming)
- Dissociation
- Multiple personalities

Older views of these phenomena in the field of psychology explain them as manifestations and evidence of the process of dissociation—where select experiences or thoughts are split off from your larger consciousness, making you unaware of them. Dr. Douglas Richards, a professor at Atlantic University in Virginia Beach with a PhD in zoology, found that dissociation was a common characteristic of several psychic experiences.[14] Dr. John F. Schumaker, a clinical psychologist and social critic, believes that hypnosis, religious and spiritual experiences, and many forms of mental illness are all created through dissociation and suggestion to avoid a reality that is perceived as threatening.[15] Attributing all of these phenomena to dissociation has its limitations. While dissociation may explain dysfunction and psychopathology, differentiation is a better means to understand the process of expanding awareness.

Examples of events in life widely attributed to dissociation that are better explained as differentiation include the experience of driving somewhere, getting to your destination, and having no recollection of the trip; watching television and not hearing someone talking to you in the same room; reading and being able to block out noise from your surroundings; or even not feeling the various articles of clothing that touch different parts of your body's skin. Such subtle sensitivities of consciousness involve a narrowing of your perceived Universe. During these processes, you block out or put into lower levels of awareness aspects of the Universe that are normally at higher levels of awareness.

Differentiation is the basic way we relate to our Universe. Differentiation is the process by which we perceive our world all day, every day, and is the fundamental way our minds work. It's always important to look at the context of the situations being examined to gain an understanding of why we see one thing and ignore another. Aspects of our Universe come into focus and go into the background along with a web of connections and associations to them that often have an emotional component. When I think of insects or bugs, I awaken many differentiations and associations that make up my relationship with these important creatures, such as my past experiences with bugs or insects, bugs in my presence at the moment, and my fears of them, to name a few. Native Americans include them as part of their family—"all my relations." I also have a friend whose wife goes ahead of him as he is mowing their lawn to warn the bugs and attempts to protect them from being harmed. Both are examples of the meaning placed on the context surrounding the experience. If I think of positive experiences in my life, I may bring positive people, places, and things into my awareness. However, when I think or concentrate on evil things, I may bring horrific perceptions into my mind. A more adequate explanation than dissociation—in which parts of the psyche are completely outside awareness—to explain selective consciousness asserts that you relate to your Universe through differentiation, since you are constantly perceiving and shifting into different levels of awareness, as you cannot attend to all aspects of your perceived Universe at any given moment.

From a perceptual point of view, dissociation is a natural process of differentiation in such situations, manifesting as threat (feeling or being threatened), boredom, and altered states. For example, when you "space out" and experience the hypnotic phenomenon of a negative hallucination (not seeing an object or person that is actually there), you actually choose not to differentiate some aspect of your perceived Universe that is somehow undesirable to you. Years ago, when I was hit head on by an automobile while driving my motorcycle, I could not recall the actual impact of my body hitting the vehicle, although I felt myself flying through the air and landing a distance away. Was my mind protecting me by forgetting the impact? Was there an involuntary recall of events? When is it choice, and when is it involuntary?

If your spirit is truly aware of everything, however, you know at some level that you are choosing what you allow yourself to experience at any moment in time. In many instances, you are still responsible for what you choose to perceive or not perceive in your Universe. For example, if I go for a walk in the woods and fail to see a pack of coyotes stalking me, my physical death may be the result. Most would agree that might be a negative experience. However, if I choose to not recall an uncomfortable interaction where a friend or family member intentionally caused me emotional pain, that might be a positive example of electing not to differentiate aspects of my experience.

MULTIPLE ASPECTS OF SELF

Hypnotic experiences as a function of both perception and the need to maximize potential may provide a more enlightening way to comprehend the phenomenon of multiple personality. Each separate personality of a person with multiple personalities perceives the world differently, and as a result, each behaves differently. Even body language and speech mannerisms change from one personality to another in such an individual. In addition, research has shown changes in eye color, allergies, and other physiological alterations have been recorded during such shifts in personality. Similar distinctions apply, if less drastically, to the multiple different aspects of a "normal" person's perceived self.

Usually as a result of traumatic experience, the new alternate personality emerges, shifting the former self to lower levels of awareness whenever that alternate personality is in command. As the person's perceived Universe is reorganized, the perceiver and the perceived fade into lower levels of awareness and remain there until another reorganization of the psyche occurs. When this process occurs, each new alternate personality or aspect of the self restricts and/or expands the perceived self, creating different abilities to recall past experience. This same process occurs for all people, on a less extreme scale. All people are integrating aspects of their perceived selves over time by reorganizing the whole as new experience affects them.

Guided hypnosis is effective in reorganizing the perceived self and Universe to such an extent that it frees the person with multiple personalities to explore past experiences in a nonthreatening manner at different levels of awareness. If such reorganization occurs, it might remove a threat and strengthen the self, eliminating the need for the perceived self to split apart to protect the overall sense of adequacy because of the characteristic ability of the human mind to reorganize itself. Dr. Eugene Taylor, who received his PhD in history and philosophy of psychology at Boston University, stated that Dr. William James, father of American psychology, in his 1896 Lowell Lectures pointed out how the phenomenon of multiple personality illustrates human potentialities:

> The fourth lecture on "Multiple Personality" argues for the existence of a growth-oriented dimension within each personality. Although psychic fragments can often develop into seemingly independent personalities, what may emerge are permanently superior dimensions not normally accessible to waking awareness.[16]

The Russian mystic Gurdjieff also claimed multiple personalities are natural aspects of all individuals. In perceptual hypnotic terms, aspects of the perceived self that were at low levels of awareness are brought into higher levels of awareness and vice versa. Some of these aspects of self in lower levels of awareness may have been lying dormant as hidden potential. By accessing multiple levels of awareness, perceptual hypnosis allows for the exploration and development of this hidden potential and of a more adequate personality. Your true self also perceives at multiple levels, many of which you don't truly understand.

THE PERCEIVED SELF

The perceived self, which is a smaller part of the perceived Universe, is also created through differentiation. The perceived self is a conceptual frame of reference, a way of defining how you view and understand self within your subjective world. In the field of hypnosis, your perceived self consists of all that you see as self, including your physical body, pain, caring, guilt, and sense of justice. Your perceived self includes everything that you experience as a part of you at any instant. This might include a child, parent, or a spouse, as well as objects, such as your house or car, completely outside your physical body. In addition, other living and nonliving aspects of the Universe may become identified as part of your self. Additional aspects of your perceived self and Universe include emotions, other living beings, and products of your imagination (including fantasies, creative works, and images). Your perceived self may also include abstract ideas.[17]

Established explanations of what happens to you when you are hypnotized contend that you dissociate from yourself. Dissociation is distancing the self from an event as it occurs, often without knowing one is taking such action. My assertion is that what occurs during hypnosis is an altering of what you focus on by choice and thereby consciously differentiate in your environment. In other words, unlike dissociation, which is a pathological explanation for a shift in awareness that one is unaware is taking place, differentiation involves a choice that one is more conscious of and is within control of the self. All aspects of hypnosis can be explained by this process of differentiation.

By engaging in hypnosis and filling in details from the Universe, you can create reorganizations of your perceived self. These reorganizations occur as you strive for adequacy in a given social context. A mother with a newborn baby may feel fulfilled in having a child but inadequate in her business career. A college student may perceive himself as an adequate student but may feel less competent as an employee starting at the bottom. Hypnosis can transform these limited views of the self.

Society pressures you to submit to its expectations and attempts to squeeze you into a narrow pattern or mold. Although at times it is necessary to narrow your perceptual possibilities to interact with others and with the Universe around you, the flexibility to expand those possibilities must never be diminished if you are to both enhance yourself and your society and maintain your self-awareness.

HOW YOU SEE YOURSELF CAN CHANGE WITH HYPNOSIS

Perceptual hypnosis can help you see yourself more accurately at a particular moment in time and remove self-imposed distortions derived from outside influences. Dr. Arthur Combs and colleagues point out that it is difficult to change perceptions of self once these perceptions have been differentiated.[18] Once the self-concept is formed, it is very resistant to change. And how you perceive yourself is incredibly important, because as Dr. Combs states: "In short, whether a person feels he is adequate or inadequate, loved or hated, strong or weak, handsome or ugly, old or young has a tremendous effect upon his behavior."[19] Often your private perception of yourself contributes to your success or failure.

Hypnosis can help you to balance a discrepancy between how you see self and how you would like to see that self. Though your total perceived Universe is always affecting you, your current level of awareness determines the view of the self in figure in your mind—what you are aware of at this moment. For example, you could be consciously upset because some unknown person has stolen a watch, pet, or other object that is important to you, while at a very low level of awareness, you really know who the culprit is. Perceptual hypnosis can remove the blinders that you wear and allow you to experience your authentic self, to discover self-identity, or to perceive new aspects of your self.

According to Dr. Combs and his colleagues, you perceive self on a continuum of adequacy to inadequacy and may feel more adequate about self in certain circumstances.[20] When you have an adequate view of yourself, you tend to see others as more adequate; whereas when you see yourself as inadequate, you tend to see others as inadequate as well.

It is interesting that clients who describe themselves as "older" often estimate others as older in age than they are, while elderly clients who consider themselves youthful often underestimate a person's actual age. Perceptions of age, beauty, and other aspects of personhood can either create barriers or foster relatedness. I recently observed two older carpenters unloading their separate work trucks of wood at the recycle center. As I approached to throw away a few boards, I overheard their conversation. The first man said: "I'm sixty years old and I love my work. I can't imagine retiring." The second man, who was tossing numerous boards like a forty year old, responded: "I'm eighty and I don't plan on retiring until my body doesn't let me work anymore." One would not have even suspected his age from his appearance or behavior. Meanwhile, a mentor of mine reported that on reaching his eightieth birthday in the fall of 2011, he was in an airport and an attendant offered him a wheelchair. He stated: "I've had a difficult time since then feeling 'youthful' for my age." An individual with an adequate personality might acknowledge diverse aspects of self and others, while others might not be able to be so flexible with their viewpoints. Hypnosis can help you to untangle distorted perceptions (such as differences between the way you perceived yourself and others in the past and the way you wished you or others were or actually were), allowing you to perceive your past self and others more accurately in the present. In our Universe, there are unlimited possibilities available.

PERCEPTUAL POINTS

- Your parents and your experiences were your first hypnotists.
- The phenomenal field is your subjective reality.
- Hypnosis is simply the process of differentiation.
- You can choose what you focus on.
- You can re-create your perceived self.

PERCEPTUAL EXERCISE

Take an important aspect of your personal world or your perceived self, and trace back the process of differentiating this important piece of your life. Try to notice every little detail of your coming to that idea or action. For example, the smell of the autumn leaves may bring a very special feeling or sensation and trigger memories of past events. Some details may seem unimportant at first. However, they may be very significant as you move forward. Notice how this idea or action unfolded in your life and became part of your world. Write this down and examine the journey. Any experience is useful for this activity, such as physical exercise, religious events, being part of a group, or choosing a movie to see.

For example, choosing a movie is a very complex experience that may otherwise seem rather simple. What is your personal history with movies? Do you watch movies alone or with others, at home or at the movie theatre? Is it a family event? Do you watch movies on certain days or at certain times? For example, on the weekend or when it is raining outside? Do you choose to watch a movie as a reward for something you did, as an escape from some difficulty in your life, or just as a way of entertaining your self, relaxing, or killing time? Do you watch a particular type of movie because someone else recommended it? Do you watch it because someone else liked it, such as a friend, relative, or coworker? Do you watch it because it is popular and everyone else has seen it? Do you watch a movie because of the feelings of excitement, comfort, or laughter it evokes within you or because the movie expresses ideas and beliefs you highly value? Tracing each aspect of what went into your choice of a movie can involve many more aspects than you recognized at the start of this exercise.

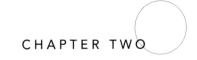

CHAPTER TWO

LIMITED PERCEPTION

If life is experience, then he who would diminish my awareness is a murderer.[21]

—*Dr. Sidney Jourard*

Although you perceive only a very narrow spectrum of objects and experiences around you while you move through your daily life, your mind is a treasure chest of potential that records far more. It is possible to tap into these hidden crevices of your mind and your self to render your daily activities and relationships more meaningful. We can look at the phenomena around us with new eyes—whether it is religion or science, media or work, family or community. We all seek the truth and often feel like we are sifting through a sea of other peoples' distortions, prejudices, or outright lies and deception. Perceiving more accurately through expanding our perceptual awareness will help us uncover some of the truths of the Universe awaiting our differentiation; this approach relies on more than the five senses to apprehend reality.

We first have to examine the sources of limited perception before we can expand awareness. At this moment you may be experiencing a narrowed and distorted perception of the world in a personally created protective bubble of existence—what I call your perceived Universe. The perceived Universe is your Universe—all that exists in your world as you experience it. It includes past experiences and resulting memories, communication with others, dreams, fantasies, and imagination. It also includes beliefs, interpretations, and desires. It may even include your computer and a friend's video game experience.

What you define as real is dependent on your perceptions, and no two people come up with the same definition of reality. Reality is subjective. For example, a client of mine who had been married for over thirty years recently lost her husband. One night while preparing to go to sleep in her bed, she perceived her husband's hand touching her face. When she told her nurse practitioner this, the clinician immediately wanted to prescribe an antipsychotic medication. In contrast, some

Nordics and Native Americans believe our ancestors watch over us as guardians. Some of my spiritual research has demonstrated that even today individuals perceive and believe that ancestors and relatives have reached out to warn or comfort them in times of distress and danger.[22] Whether the widow's encounter with her husband was a hallucination or not depends on your perceived Universe. What is real to you is what is in your perceptual awareness. These slices of experience are all aspects of your perceived Universe—true or not.

FAILURE TO DIFFERENTIATE

How does differentiation appear in our lives on a daily basis? How do we use it without even being aware of it? What effect is the process of differentiating having on us? We don't realize that we are constantly distorting our reality to create a perceived Universe that doesn't conflict with our current views. If you are finding time to stay physically fit or advance your career or personal development, for example, when you interact with others who are unable to follow in your footsteps, you might find verbal messages of discouragement and untrue facts being lodged at you: "I have to put food on the table for my family, so I don't have time to work out." "Don't quit your day job." "Lawyers are crooks." These are broad statements based on black and white thinking that can limit a person's perceptions. The last statement or truism leaves out the fact that some lawyers have helped defend people against powerful and unscrupulous individuals, for example. A father might talk his son out of being a lawyer because the profession would outdo his perceived view of his own personal and professional power. He tells his son there are too many lawyers, lawyers are not liked, and lawyers are corrupt, while secretly the father does not want his son to have a more influential job in the community than he himself has. What aspects of the Universe the son chooses to differentiate in his experience of becoming a lawyer determines whether he follows his goal or abandons it. We may not realize how dependent our life-altering decisions are on the process of differentiation.

EVERYDAY HYPNOSIS

In your everyday experiences you may encounter forms of hypnosis—subtle manipulations from others and outright instances of mind control—that limit your worldview. And these influences have a great impact on how the self is formed. The most optimal condition for one's personal growth would be to receive encouragement and support when trying to reach for a new level in life. When learning something new, children need some direction and a stress-free environment. When a child encounters an adult who really cares for him or her, a parent or teacher whose attention says: "You're the apple of my eye," or "I believe in you," that child shines. Wouldn't it be nice if adults could experience similar positive conditions when they attempt change or growth? But unfortunately, it's not always the case. If one breaks from family tradition, for example, the change in behavior can be met with resistance or negativity. Those who do not welcome change might ignore your personal growth or accomplishments. Some may attribute another's success to a false source or downplay it. For instance, a person might say a figure skater is someone with a natural gift who didn't require extensive hours of training to explain away his or her own lack of achievement. There are numerous ways that others can try to maintain the status quo in your mind, to impose limits, by ignoring the truth and leading you to misperceive. If you are affected by these efforts of others, or even allow them to influence you without being fully conscious of the dynamic, you can consider yourself hypnotized. If you are wondering if you are resistant to change in your own life, you might ask yourself how you react to others who are changing or have made changes. It is often easier to see our attitudes reflected in the ways we treat others. Do you encourage others when they are thinking of making changes in their lives? Does it make you feel anxious to hear about someone taking a risk? Does your mind go to a negative place or a hopeful place?

Institutions attempt to instill fear, guilt, and shame to promote a particular viewpoint. Often you fear reprisals for ethically speaking out. Fearful of losing your job, income, and security, you might act unethically or ignore your basic spiritual values. In such situations, you are not truly free to perceive alternatives in life or to determine personal truth in an ever-changing Universe. Your mind is often filled with irrelevant facts and knowledge as you are shown what to perceive directly—in social, political, or religious settings—rather than about how to use your own powers of observation. You are often distracted from the truth. This can lead you to act in ways that don't feel right to you, and even to compromise your values. Paul Tillich, a German-American Christian existentialist philosopher and theologian, defined guilt as ". . . the pollution of the soul by the material realm or by demonic powers."[23] This striving for security or protection at all costs against perceived threats creates a self-imposed prison and limits your ability to reach your full potential. Perceptual hypnosis helps create a shield that can deflect such influences. For example, one can imagine the ocean waves bringing a healing and relaxing energy into your body and removing any negative influences that block your growth. In other words, hypnosis can help you to organize your psyche and to become aware of the many influences that affect your thoughts, feelings, and bodily awareness through training your perceptual awareness.

You often spontaneously enter everyday hypnosis without being aware of it. Everyone is hypnotized at some point in this sense. For example, if you look at your viewpoints and opinions and trace them back to their origins, you will sometimes be amazed at the results. You may find that you have mindlessly taken on beliefs and perceptions simply because others asserted that they were true.

In other words, when everyday hypnosis occurs, it derives from external forces that have often hypnotized you without any formal hypnotic procedure being involved. Experiences we have had, statements made to us assertively by other people, and ideas passed on unconsciously from earlier generations create fact out of fiction and become your world.

Without an accurate understanding of how hypnosis works in everyday life, you can be a victim of others' desires and influences. Everyday hypnotism is at work in all areas of society—computer spam, political slogans, and movie posters, to name a few. Those who are aware of how to manipulate your internal experiences and change how you perceive things in order to shape your behavior can use this knowledge to influence you for their personal benefit rather than your own.

Facing your fears may feel like walking through a sheet of glass. You imagine your life will fall apart or you will shatter as you experience a threat to your present perceived self and Universe. You might imagine that the glass will crumble and scatter into many pieces on the ground. In the end, you will often find that you have survived unharmed, with maybe a few scratches after facing your fears and dealing with imagined threats. What has actually shattered is a distorted perception from your past experience that you had the courage to break away from. On the other side of the fence, mentors, loving family and friends, and teachers often help us differentiate empowering aspects of the Universe that move us toward health and growth. In the movie, *The Lion King*, Rafiki, the wise old baboon, and Nala, Simba's childhood sweetheart, awakened in Simba forgotten memories that allowed him to change his damaged sense of self and return to Pride Rock to defend his family and regain his true sense of self. Refiki reminded Simba that his father was still alive by saying, "He lives in you." Refiki's statement evoked in Simba a vision of his father, Mufasa, telling Simba that he had forgotten him, and in forgetting his father, Simba had forgotten who he himself was. This vision caused a change in Simba, who then gained a connection with his true self and was led to see past events more accurately and to uncover the truth of his father's death.

THREAT AND IMPOSED MIND CONTROL

Threat and imposed mind control are significant methods to narrow or distort our perceptual awareness. Threat is an external influence that has occurred throughout human history as a natural phenomenon among humans. Threat can arise from the natural world in the form of disasters or predatory animals, from the human sphere in the form of violence or competition. Each of us has had an encounter with danger or trauma, or simply experienced feeling unsafe.

Until you fully understand that you and no one else can create and control your thinking, you will never be in control of your life. You will continue to be vulnerable to others' desires and wishes. You can take responsibility for your perceptual awareness, however, through using hypnosis. You can stop blaming others for your personal thoughts, feelings, and bodily experiences. You are the creator of your perceived Universe and an explorer in a broader Universe where many aspects still remain for you to discover.

A perceived threat can be created by distorted thinking and is actually quite common. Such a subjective view of the world is created when the environment is believed in an unrealistic sense to have the potential to harm. Escalating arms races between nations is an extreme version of this. Antisocial and paranoid ideations are also examples of perceived threats created by distorted thinking. In smaller ways, this can happen in relationships, but can have great impact if misunderstood. A client of mine relayed how she was often upset with her husband, who did not pay attention to her after his workday's end. Instead, he spent endless hours on repairs and upkeep of their house. She felt his actions implied she was unimportant or their marriage was insignificant. When asked about his actions, he responded that he had suffered a heart attack a few years prior and wanted his wife and son to have security if anything happened to him, so he was making sure the house was well taken care of. My client's view of her husband's behavior as distancing himself from her was distorted. It was not that he didn't care about his wife or family but rather that he cared quite a bit, enough to sacrifice his own enjoyment for their security.

Some individuals differentiate aspects of the Universe that don't exist for the other; for example, spiritual experiences that are reported can be a threat for other people because they shake up a preconceived world view. For example, a client of mine relayed an event that happened while watching his father-in-law dying. His father-in-law was in and out of consciousness, and when he finally came back to conscious awareness, he told his son: "I just talked to your sister. They are waiting for me. I don't understand. . . . She had two little girls and they were calling me 'Grandpa.'" The son-in-law burst into tears. His wife, who'd died a few years earlier, had had two miscarriages that they had not told anyone about. For the son-in-law, that was validation of an afterlife; for a fundamentalist, it could represent a threat to an established belief system. A challenge to one's world view can be perceived as threatening. This type of reaction to threat is curable through hypnosis with a perceptual emphasis.

Invitations to expand one's perceived Universe with new ideas can be distressing to some. Unfamiliar concepts may be received as a negation of one's current world view, in a form of black and white thinking. With the increased anxiety that arises with new ideas and experiences, a threatened person may revert to a more simplistic way of conceptualizing his world: There is only right and wrong; it is not within my scope of experience, so it must be wrong. The perceived threat typically elicits this type of adverse reaction.

Threat narrows and restricts the flexibility of your perceptual awareness and limits your differentiation of aspects of the Universe. For example, an individual can contribute to your perception of threat by magnifying selected incidents. A person who knows you want to learn to ski tells you about the horrific skiing accident of a family friend. The person who tries to create these perceptions may enhance his or her need for adequacy through limiting your choices and activities, and in turn increase your feelings of inadequacy through fears of negative outcomes. Some individuals manipulate your perspective by creating a threat or distorting reality for political, religious, or economic gain. History has shown that realities perceived by a population majority are often distorted and incorrect, affected by the political beliefs and culture of a particular time period. For example, at one time the majority of Americans believed slavery was acceptable. Even as recently as the twentieth century, Native Americans have been denied the right to vote. Penobscot Indian Charles N. Shay, a D-day veteran, who dodged bullets on Omaha Beach and miraculously remained unharmed as a medic in World War II and later in the Korean War, was denied the right to vote despite being decorated as a war hero. He was not treated like a full citizen of the United States.[24] When he dressed in uniform with all his medals and walked with his family into the town hall in Old Towne, Maine, to vote in a local election, he was told by the officials: "Idiots don't vote." Native Americans did not get the right to vote in Maine until 1954, and for some local and state elections, it took until 1967 to obtain that right. Yet the likelihood is quite high that he had saved the lives of distant members of these officials' families. History contains both progress from the past and limitations from the past. Those limitations are forced on the populace by the masses adhering to rigid concepts and misperceived and distorted aspects of the Universe. However, Shay's mother, whose letter to the president of the United States helped gain the Native Americans' right to vote in Maine, helps us understand that individuals can alter group distortions.

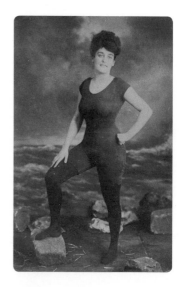

A great example of this is the **picture** of Annette Kellerman. She was promoting a woman's right to wear a fitted, one-piece bathing suit in 1907. However, she was later arrested for indecency. How are freedoms such as this being infringed upon today?

No one is entirely free of the cultural influences and control that affect individual thoughts, limit personal options, and sculpt behavior. Cultural experiences create consensus thinking among groups;

Annette Kellerman, 1907. Exercising women's right to wear a fitted bathing suit.

these constructs may be interpreted as fundamental truths, which may restrict some people from opening up to other possibilities and limit their relationships to reality. Drs. Snygg and Combs posited this notion when they stated: "What is accepted as fact in any culture is no more than what the majority of its important people believe to be true."[25]

TAKING AWAY RESPONSIBILITY—DISTORTING PERCEPTION

External forces that impede our thoughts and actions can alter the meaning of our lives. Our place in the world becomes further removed from our truer self. Dr. Ian Stevenson was a psychiatrist who studied reincarnation at the University of Virginia. He pointed out that individuals in Western society are losing an ability to take responsibility for their lives and actions. He maintained that religion provides excuses for people's lack of responsibility by promoting ideas such as predestination, or by implying that Christ's crucifixion removes any obligation to make restitution for one's own sins. Alongside religion, science provides theories of both chance and evolution to explain experience, presented as beyond individual control and thus beyond individual responsibility.[26] Medication originally created to help people heal has become an exploitive multimillion dollar business that peddles addictive substances called "psychotropics." Is advertising not influencing people through hypnotic communication? For example, pills to treat illnesses caused by an unhealthy lifestyle obviously aren't curing the source of the problem; quite frequently, pharmaceuticals are used to avoid making a change to a healthier lifestyle, which can still lead to premature deaths or disabilities. We are telling children not to do street drugs, but advertisements in magazines and on television send messages continuously that a pill will solve all your problems. Producers of one medication emphasize that you can feel more adequate about your social life with their pill, while minimizing the side effects—that your feelings may be numbed out and you might even become sexually dysfunctional. Prescription medications have now become an addiction problem for youth and are being illegally sold on the streets.

There are some exceptional professionals in the field of psychology, like the deceased Dr. Kevin McCready, a clinical psychologist from Fresno, California, who created a psychological clinic that treated individuals for mental illness without medication. I was able to participate in this very rare experience during my doctoral training and found it invaluable later in my career. Often patients in mental health settings complain about being prescribed excessive medications and want alternative ways to overcome their difficulties. Research has shown that about one out of three persons do not benefit from psychiatric medications. There are some psychiatrists, however, who work to expand knowledge in medicine, such as Dr. Peter Breggin, who wrote *Toxic Psychiatry* and examined the negative aspects of individuals taking medication for psychological problems. This is not to disregard psychiatric medicines prescribed responsibly by many professionals. A colleague of mine, Dr. Robert Kaladish of Amherst, New Hampshire, utilizes psychiatric medicine and naturopathic holistic medicine to help people with mental illnesses.

Another way that outside influences can distort your perception is through money. The use of money as a means of controlling and conditioning people has restricted some peoples' perceptual awareness in drastic ways and unnaturally limited their differentiation. Society has become a marketplace, and the dollar for some has become the god of modern times. A community based on rewards and punishments has been created through a monetary system that perpetuates itself and vigorously defends the injustices it imposes, for example, by limiting opportunities and access to resources. Some individuals cannot buy homes, go to college, or receive proper medical treatment due to lack of funds.

The question is, are you allowing others to influence your thoughts, feelings, and behaviors? If so, you might unwittingly let yourself be manipulated. Or, if you are perceptually aware, you might try to resist such influences. This requires you to educate yourself, to make choices about what you're exposed to, to discern and read between the lines. It can be difficult to discern the truth. As Professor Joel Fort MD at the University of California at Berkeley has explained:

> We are further confused by the progressive debasement of language by the media, press agents, advertisers, and politicians. Evil has become good; war has become peace; and mediocre is thought of as outstanding. Lies, omissions, distortions, and euphemisms have become institutionalized. As Frank Lloyd Wright said: "2 percent of the people think; 8 percent think that they think; and 90 percent would be caught dead before thinking."[27]

Mediocre people maintain the status quo. They have been robbed of their true potential. And they see other people as objects to be used as commodities to advance their financial position. Money is placed above ethics. "Executives of mediocrity" wash their hands of any ethical values other than how to advance the financial position of their organizations or themselves. They compete with each other using gender, age, race, cars, houses, and salaries as evidence of superior or inferior status, very rarely perceiving what is actually wrong with the social world. As Dr. K E. Boulding, economist and social psychologist who graduated from Oxford University and taught at University of Colorado at Boulder for years, asserted: "Every craft which has a self-conscious image of itself in the minds of its members is to some extent a conspiracy against the public."[28]

Other ways that external forces can control or limit the functioning of your mind include:

- **Contradictory laws.** For example, an eighteen-year-old can fight in a war but cannot consume alcoholic beverages.
- **Science that is biased.** Experts explain away new research on near-death experiences as just distortions of brain chemicals and pharmaceutical drugs. Many scientific discoveries have been costly to doctors who are threatened, ostracized, and ignored because their accomplishments changed the status quo, such as circulation of blood in the body, discovery of bacteria, washing hands before surgery, neuroplasticity—the discovery that we can grow new brain cells at any age and nerves can connect to different parts of the brain and create new pathways, even in older adults.
- **Economic obstacles and restrictions to freedom.** A historical example is the discovery in the 1800s of hypnosis as a technique to remove pain during surgery. Instead of promoting the understanding of this knowledge to heal your self with inner resources, primary effort was placed on external changes through chemical anesthesia. These drugs require continual payment for services. Self-hypnosis requires mental abilities that, once mastered, are your own indefinitely, without any further cost.

PERCEPTUAL POINTS

- We've all been hypnotized without agreeing to any formal hypnotic procedure.
- To expand perceptual awareness, we need to identify the external influences that limit our perception.
- Significant individuals, institutions, and past experiences distort our perceptual awareness.
- Through the process of differentiation, we can remove these restrictions to our personal growth.

PERCEPTUAL EXERCISE

This activity asks you to identify limits to your perceptual awareness, restrictions to your mind, and to question facts you may have accepted with limited evidence. As you look honestly at yourself, a new way of perceiving and living your life can begin to unfold. Identify one personal or historical event in which a distortion of perception came to light. Journal the unfolding of this change in awareness and perspective and what took place from beginning to end.

List experiences where you found the truth to be contrary to what you previously believed or perceived. This experience might have happened upon meeting a person who surprised you somehow. It may have occurred when your plans to do something were not fulfilled. Or it may have been a time when you impressed or disappointed yourself.

List the various sources of distortions your mind created before being confronted with the new truth.

Journal how your change in perceptions and/or behaviors created a new situation—how your life was altered.

For example, here is a brief summary of an event that changed perspective.

1. Experience that Changed Perception: A person has an out-of-body experience and sees a dead crow on a roof. The person was unable to see the crow on the roof in any other known way.
2. Previous Distorted Perception: This person was not supposed to be able to experience things out of his body nor observe the crow.
3. Effect on Your Perceived Self or Personal World: Profound change in the way the person interacts with others and reacts to death issues.

SELF-HYPNOSIS PRACTICE

Imagine that you are walking on a beach. You feel the dry warm granules of sand between your toes. You see the blue sky. Feel the soft, gentle breeze on your face and skin. Hear the ocean waves rhythmically wash onto the beach. Inhale the ocean air and feel a deep sense of relaxation entering your body, mind, and spirit. See the sea gulls gliding through the air and hear their noises as they are moving about. See the sunlight glittering off the ocean water. And now walk down to where the water and the land meet.

You imagine a gentle little wave splashes up and bubbles on your feet and ankles, bringing a warm wave of relaxation throughout your entire body. It feels so good to relax and let go. As each wave comes in, you feel this wave of relaxation. As each wave goes out, you feel the chains, blocks, and obstacles to your self-growth falling away and being carried out to the ocean, into the depths where they are disintegrated and can no longer harm you. You can do this for as long as you like. Your true potential is released as your restrictions and limitations are removed. Practice this exercise daily.

You can take this exercise one level deeper by going to a body of water—pond, lake, stream, river—experiencing its calming and clearing qualities by stepping into the water. You may want to notice the life connected to this body of water. See the deer drinking by the water's edge on the bank. Notice the insects particular to this body of water. The plants that are present hold a special place in the setting. Notice your own connections in your life and deepen them. Water is very soothing and life-affirming. You might begin to observe how these connections expand your positive experiences of the Universe in your life, allow you to identify with others, to notice diverse perceptions and be open to new experiences different from your past. You may want to take a swim to wash away and release some of the weight or burden of old beliefs and limitations.

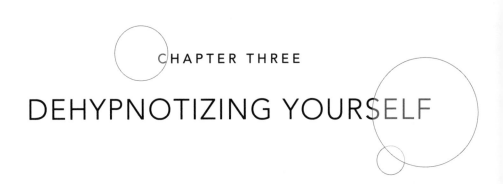

CHAPTER THREE

DEHYPNOTIZING YOURSELF

Every conflict over truth is in the last analysis just the same old struggle over the existence and immortality of the soul.[29]

—Dr. Otto Rank

To understand how perceptual hypnosis can be used as a powerful tool to increase and develop your spiritual awareness, you must begin awakening—dehypnotizing—yourself basically from external influences and false learnings. I recommend you develop perceptually expanding activities using a process that I call **perceptual hypnosis**. This process helps you fight off negative influences, such as mind control and generational patterns you want to transcend, that block your human potential and can shape your thoughts and behavior every day. These negative influences naturally occur as you open up to new experiences and expand your Universe.

Understanding and applying the theory of perceptual hypnosis presented in this book will allow you to perceive reality more clearly and accurately, and connect to the hitherto unrecognized invisible influences all around you. You will grow to identify the more subtle influences in your life that remain unobserved. In this way you will be able to express new dimensions of yourself, including your spiritual potential. When you perceive more accurately, you will connect with the spiritual world, in whatever way is acceptable to you, more deeply and genuinely. You may begin to see things in a new and different way than before. You may see how some random events are not so random. You may develop a deeper connection with nature. You may notice how facts are not always correct.

By "hypnotize" or "dehypnotize" I mean to awaken from that which is unrealized and open up to a full consciousness that contains possibilities you may have been unknowingly taught to disregard or to believe do not exist. Unfortunately, the popular belief is that hypnosis puts you to sleep, takes over your will, or influences you in a negative way. This could not be further from the truth. Instead, this broader way of experiencing the world can alter your perceived Universe, making it more flexible and accurate by revealing new aspects of the actual Universe that have previously remained unseen or been at low levels of awareness.

A hypnotic trance is nothing more than an alteration of your perceptual awareness brought about by narrowing or expanding your ability to differentiate aspects of the Universe. Examples of narrowing your perceptions include studying for a test, listening to your body or inner experience and are found in moments of an intense experience, such as becoming one with a musical instrument, an intimate other, or a sports activity. Examples of expanding your world include discovering new species of animals, life on another planet, and that our bodies and minds can develop new abilities and functions well into old age. As such, altered states of awareness and trance are simply a matter of differentiation—shifts in perceptual awareness.

Trance is defined in the Merriam-Webster Dictionary as "a state in which you are not aware of what is happening around you because you are thinking of something else"[30] (by permission Merriam-Webster, Springfield, MA. www.meriam-webster. com/dictionary/trance. 2015.). In trance you bring some aspects of your world into focus while you ignore other aspects of the world. In other words, you differentiate.

ALTERING OUR LIMITED CONSCIOUSNESS

You can choose to access your inner capabilities spiritually and expand your life or remain in a restricted mode that can render you a victim of outside influences and your internal distortions. As is true for most people, you utilize only a very small fraction of the total undeveloped abilities within you. Many have expressed this idea throughout history. James Wyckoff, author of the biography of Dr. Franz Anton Mesmer, who was a German physician and the father of hypnosis, is one of numerous writers who have spoken about the common lack of awareness of the Universe and about external influences that distort individual views of it. For example, Wyckoff stated: "Great teachers and religious leaders have appeared throughout history to reassert what has already been known, to begin again the effort to help man raise himself out of his hypnotic sleep to a more real reality."[31] This real reality includes a spiritual awareness in our lives. Spiritual awareness takes in all that exists. It includes that which remains invisible to most but exists nonetheless, including paranormal events and healing through subtle energy techniques. For example, ask a body of water to assist you in releasing the false blocks you have created and developed, and that prevented you from experiencing the freedom you deserved. More discussion on this subject is in Chapters 9 and 10.

DIVERSE PERCEPTUAL AWARENESS

Perceptual awareness is a clear and enduring interior experience that is often manifested in diverse ways in the world around you. You have many ways of understanding your world and the Universe. Even if you are not primarily a visual learner and learn better through hearing (auditory sensory input) or touch (tactile sensory input), at the foundation of any learning approach is a fundamental perceptual awareness that simultaneously stimulates your mind and the multiple senses that contribute to your experience. Dr. James Esdaile, a Scottish surgeon, did not find it necessary for the individuals' eyes to be open when being hypnotized. He had them close their eyes to remove distractions during hypnosis. He noted that blind men are just as easily mesmerized as others. In fact, being hypnotized—becoming perceptually aware—like learning is enhanced by input to multiple senses that need not include vision.

Another example of the various ways that different people perceive is how a blind person may "see" through touch. Bishop George Berkeley, an Anglo-Irish philosopher, pointed out the uniqueness of perceptual awareness as he stated of the blind in 1709: that a man born blind, being made to see, would at first have no idea of distance by sight: the sun and stars, the remotest objects as well as the nearer, would all seem to be in his eye, or rather in his mind.[32]

Further George Berkeley explained the diversity of ways of perceiving:

The truth is, the things I see are so very different and heterogeneous from the things I feel that the perception of the one would never have suggested the other to my thoughts, or enabled me to pass the least judgment thereon, until I had experienced their connexion [sic].[33]

Our perceptual awareness seems to affect how and what aspects of the Universe we are able to perceive, for better or for worse. Dr. Leo Buscaglia said that the human limitations in the power of perception can be illustrated by watching a group of blindfolded people all wearing no clothes trying to identify one another.[34] Behind most spoken or written words are meanings founded in limitless possibilities unique to each individual, which is enhanced with a qualitative research process that seeks out individuality rather than suppressing it, while recognizing the many commonalities we share in human experience. For example, while we can easily in the north comprehend a freshly fallen snow, it is much more difficult to recognize that each snowflake is completely unique and different, just as each person's fingerprints.

Hypnotists have always known about the potential power an image has after your attention is focused and your body is relaxed. Such images create a reorganization of your perceived Universe, altering your internal experience in both higher and lower levels of awareness. With few exceptions, specific external aspects remain at higher levels of awareness. In this case, a hypnotist need not assist you in entering an altered level of awareness—simply sitting down in a relaxing chair and centering your attention on the television does!

DEHYPNOTIZING CAN BE PAINFUL

Dehypnotizing yourself—changing your perceptual awareness—may cause you to experience what is referred to as "the dark night of the soul," a process during which the meaning of your life is drastically altered, your world appears shattered, and your past and present are transformed as your perceived meaning of what is true or real is permanently changed. Entering this process is a transition or passage necessary for furthering spiritual growth, development, and transformation. When I do research in phenomenology, the first step is to observe something without preconceptions, bias, and assumptions. I then am able to remove illusions with an openness to new experiences, as if clearing the slate or wiping the white board clean of past memories and associations to open to a greater meaningfulness in the now. This illumination and deeper sense of purpose or connectedness occurs when we destroy what limits and restricts our perceptual awareness from our past internal mislearnings and outside influences. An example would be that you may not be the only one influencing your body, mind, and spirit. Many famous writers felt they were channeling knowledge from greater sources, and some doctors of dentistry, psychology, and psychiatry have examined what they believed were cases of possession.

When we deepen our views, changes occur in how we interact with others, conduct ourselves, and in the meaning we place on our lives. We may come to believe that our behaviors and thoughts are seen by God or other entities, or that we may have past or future lives, and that there are other realities, viewpoints, and possibilities other than our own that are relevant and important.

The paranormal and spiritual experiences discussed in this chapter point to changes that take place inside persons either prior to or as a result of their experiences. Inner experiences can ultimately create your external reality. Many different sources have pointed out this perceptual fact. A vivid, creatively imagined internal world has a way of manifesting in your external world, blurring the boundaries between them.

On this point, a number of psychologists have agreed, according to authors A. A. Sheikh and C. S. Jordon, that ". . . experiencing something in imagery can be considered to be in many essential ways psychologically equivalent to experiencing the thing in actuality."[35] The Bible speaks about a thought of something being as real as is an action itself. Your imagination gives you the power to create an internal or inner vision of your potential.

Research in neuropsychology indicates that imagining physical movement simulates activation of your nervous system—as if a movement is actually occurring. If you imagine something, such as a success, your body and being often respond as if it has actually occurred. This data corresponds to how you might immediately attempt to counter any imaginings of a negative event with positive thoughts for fear that the event might really manifest in life because of negative thoughts.

The power of your mind is supported by further research showing that perceptual thought can influence growth of plants. Further, during an experiment in undergraduate school, I witnessed a fellow student project an image of a rose onto photographic film in a dark room. Others have demonstrated this skill.[36, 37]

Dr. James Woodard summarizes a group of childhood experiences that later become relevant in an unfolding of the sense of self in spiritual and paranormal experience:

> Since the child assumes thought to be inseparable from its object, confuses thoughts and things, identifies names with the things named, takes dreams to be external and material, and in a great many other ways confuses the subjective with the objective and the self with the not-self, it must be evident that he can scarcely escape the feeling of magical participation on the part of thought and self with the events that occur in the external world. . . . and the child is of a long time under the naïve conception that his thoughts are open to others.[38]

You can learn from children as well as adults. Childhood innocence emanates wisdom, since children are not completely socially conditioned and have not yet cognitively reframed everything they see and think to fit in a particular box the way many adults have. Questions that result from observing children and that are worth considering are:

- Just how far does individual influence extend?
- What is part of the self and what is not part of the self?
- How accurate is the average person's perceptual awareness of the actual Universe?

I know that all of my past experiences and knowledge have led me to this point in my life, and that yours have led you to where you are now. Even my least appealing experiences had a part in bringing about greater understanding and expansion of my perceptual awareness. I hope that this book helps bridge a gap between religion, spirituality, and hypnosis for you. I hope I can dispel fears created by external influences that may have already impacted your differentiating, so that you are able to come closer to an expansion of your perceptual awareness or a validation of similar experiences. You are beginning to open to a more flexible perceived Universe. Such life-changing events are often initiated by some unforeseen trauma or misfortune or happenings. Common examples are death of loved ones, severe injuries or accidents, abuse or crime victimization, war, natural disasters, or loss of jobs and homes. Often clients come into therapy when such an event or tragedy moves them from an otherwise acceptable lifestyle to a daily functioning that is no longer validating. Their lives may seem confined or like nothing makes sense any more. A person may feel that there is no God or that God has abandoned them, that life has no purpose, there is an unknowing or uncertainty and meaninglessness filling their perceptions and awareness. There is comfort nowhere and everything seems unfamiliar. In this stage the person is letting go of false perceptions, which is a really painful process. There are diverse and new possibilities entering your awareness. An encounter with some unusual experience may occur that alters your perceived understanding of how your life unfolds. You may feel separate and different or set apart from the rest of your friends, family, and community, even when it does not appear that way on the outside to others in your life. You might feel totally alone, even among others. Examples of unusual experiences can be visits from ancestors, ghosts and entities appearing, synchronistic events that cannot be explained, grasped, or defined in a normal or casual way. You feel like your world is falling apart—you are no longer able to maintain your old patterns of living. You feel like no one or nothing can make you feel whole; common thoughts, beliefs, and behaviors are no longer beneficial as they were for you in the past, leaving you feeling empty or hollow. You might feel stuck with no way out. Examples may be old beliefs that turn out to not be true, medications that don't solve the problem, or people from other races or countries who perceive things differently and expand your knowledge by proving some of your old beliefs false.

Eventually, new growth means that you begin to identify with others in a more connected, richer, and deeper way. Spiritually you expand your sense of self so that you see in a new way. Old barriers are no longer valid. Distance may not interfere with your perceptual awareness of another person who is emotionally close or important to you in some way. You may become aware of your intricate connections to all of life.

For example, a woman whose sister died would see her sister at night in her dreams and tell family members that her sister had spoken with her. The family did not believe her, and of course their negative comments began to hurt the girl's faith in her dreams of her sister. Then, on one particular night, the sister told her that she would prove that she is real and these dreams are not just her imagination. The sister took the dreamer into a room where there was a famous actor, who was thought to be alive at the time. He turned around and greeted the dreamer and told her that he was killed by his girlfriend. The girl woke and told her family what she had dreamed in the morning. Later that day, news and television reported that the actor was discovered dead in his home. The family still didn't believe this research subject, and she became quiet as her mother threatened to force her to see a psychiatrist.

Yet another example involves a man riding on his motorcycle in the early evening. At that time, he had a vision and heard his thoughts in his mind say that his girlfriend was visiting with an older man ("Mike") who had a crush on her. He noticed the time, and the next day told his girlfriend, who accused him of spying on her or reading her journal. She had indeed seen Mike that very evening. These are examples of how conventional time and space are transcended by those who are more connected to those they care about.

In finding your connectedness, you begin to see that your actions can have far-reaching consequences, even when they are initially seen as benign or insignificant. An example would be that my great-grandfather and grandmother from Boston, Massachusetts, in the 1600s more than likely did not realize that from them would descend many doctors, lawyers, and captains in the Revolutionary War, among others. You begin to perceive the invisible links, and the circle of life takes on a greater meaning.

Your expanding awareness alters your personal world. Positive experiences may melt away the limits you place on yourself from past false learning or interactions with others. You become more expansive and positive, which opens you to a greater Universe. For example, rather than seeing aliens as a contradiction of your religion, you realize God is the creator of all things and, therefore, accept new and unusual findings in your life as enhancing rather than as threatening.

On occasion when lifting weights, I will accidentally put the peg of weight indicator on a Nautilus machine slightly higher than I realized and unknowingly prove to myself that I can lift more weight than I thought I could. Another example of a person expanding his personal world through breaking down false limits is professional baseball player James Anthony Abbott, who was able to become a pitcher despite being born without a right hand. He played for the California Angels, the New York Yankees, the Chicago White Sox, and the Milwaukee Brewers from 1989 to 1999. Similarly, you can see how an experience of being weaker can become the impetus for growth and lead a person to become stronger by discovering how to stand up to another. So in many ways, we can expand our experiences and overcome our limits with a new perceptual view.

Solid evidence has also enhanced human understanding and expanded perceptions. For instance, over time, DNA testing by forensic psychologists and scientists has led to the discovery that many men in jail are innocent of the charges that put them behind bars. Through new knowledge and self-growth, people expand their Universes and their ability to differentiate new aspects of themselves or others.

William James, father of American psychology and Harvard psychologist, studied altered states of consciousness, parapsychology, and spirituality. He pointed out that some individuals would be fascinated by the simplest aspects of hypnosis, while others would deny its benefits, even if it brought someone back from the dead. He perceived consciousness as a stream of water and an undivided multiplicity never able to be dissected or understood by a simple element extracted from the stream.[39] The questions perceptual hypnosis asks are:

- How accurate is your awareness of the Universe right now?
- How can you change your mind to see the world more accurately?

In order to see accurately, you need to understand the context of the situation. The more accurately you can perceive the Universe, the less likely you will be negatively influenced by events in your life and the more likely you can understand events for what they fundamentally represent. You will be less likely to take things inappropriately, out of context, or be fooled by others who try to influence your perceptions and behavior. From this more holistic perspective, you will be able to function from a place of increased strength and wisdom. So let's look at an example of a case study where consciousness was expanded with new and unusual spiritual or paranormal experiences.

CASE STUDY OF SHADOW FIGURES

For this thirty-three-year-old single woman of French and Abenaki descent, medication and cognitive-behavioral therapy was ineffective. Her spiritual thoughts and experiences were a combination of Native American, Pagan, and Christian traditions, best described as a mystical orientation. She had three master degrees in psychology, education, and the arts. She had been in mental health treatment for six years. She had gone through several therapists, tried multiple techniques, and had tried numerous medications to no avail. She eventually stopped sharing her symptoms with others. As long as this participant could remember, she had had negative experiences with shadow figures whisking by her during the day in her home and at night in her bedroom. They'd begun when she was very young, as she reported various entities often tried to influence her to hurt herself. She described these beings from visual experiences during interactions with them. This participant supposed that these entities were unable to act in the material or physical world on their own behalf and, therefore, mentally attempted to persuade her to hurt herself for them.

This participant described these shadow figures passing by her as dark and like blobs that are able to change appearance and shapes. Sometimes she would see them out of the corner of her eyes as whisking by her. At other times they would appear like blobs. Sometimes they would take the shape of a person and have eyes and a mouth.

She often felt a hostile or adversarial presence in her room and always experienced shadow figures on her walls. She felt those black shadow figures as an impinging doom. This participant described these black shadow figures as located more on the south side of her room across from her bed. When she woke up at night and her room was dark (there were no light sources in her room), she always perceived a part of her room as much darker and blacker than anything else. She stated: "I can see in the dark and through the darkness in my room, but not through those dark shadow figures or entities. They are like a solid black blob lacking any light." She described the shadow figures in a dark room as blacker than black.

At one point she had awakened in the middle of the night and had gotten out of bed and was able to see in her room until this blackness entered her and took her over, and she could not move or see. It was as if she had gone blind and was paralyzed. She then felt this energy leave her, urinated on her bedroom floor, and could suddenly see again in the dark. This incident was both embarrassing and had never happened to her before or since that night. This incident frightened her so much she turned to spiritual people for help, as she felt that it was an external force and not something that came from within. One doctor had described it as "a neurological malfunction." A cognitive behavioral therapist stated she must have fantasized or hallucinated this experience. She felt this experience as an external force that entered her being and made it impossible for her to see or move, while she remained conscious of this experience happening, as if trapped in a cage.

On another occasion, when she was eleven years old, she was standing at the tree in the front yard of her uncle's house. It was by the swing set. She was standing with her left hand on a rope to the swing at waist level, facing the forest. Her uncle's two German shepherds (Blackjack and Shadow) were there. Blackjack was facing her and Shadow was beside her, facing the forest. She was looking down at Blackjack and patting Shadow on the back. It was just after dinner and her uncle had gone for a walk. A dark shadow passed in front of her, and her vision faded to black. She didn't know how much time had passed, but her vision came back and the two dogs were facing her and growling, with their teeth bared. She started to shake with fear. Her aunt came to the door and yelled at the dogs. They left and she stood there frozen for a while. Her aunt asked if she was okay and she answered, "Yes." She got on her skateboard and went home.

The black shadow figures that appeared in her room or on her south walls moved very slowly and calculatingly and would glide up, down, and across her walls. This participant described those shadow figures on her walls as a very detrimental energy or giving her a gloomy feeling. She described her apparitions as creepy, fearful, and distressing to her. After these terrifying experiences, she felt shook up and out of harmony with herself, as if suddenly, for no reason, she didn't like herself. She felt like she needed to withdraw or retreat, but there was nowhere to go. It was as if someone was stalking or hunting her, but she had no real evidence that anyone was there so that she could act upon her inner impressions or prove them to others. At one point, at age twenty-two, an invisible force dragged her off her bed and pulled her hair. Something invisible slapped the back of her head, but she saw nothing she could describe except the sensations that she felt. She went to stay with a friend after these incidents of pulling and physical slapping for over a week because she was so scared.

These shadow figure experiences created so much fear in her that her body went on high alert and would become immobile, as if she could not move, with a desire to disappear. These experiences frightened her so much that on two occasions she urinated on herself in her room. She smelled a stench that turned her stomach and felt like it passed through her. This putrid smell had no logical source or place of origin. It would make her frightened when her bed would rock and move without any apparent cause. She described that unreasonable fear totally taking over her mind and attention as she froze or became rigid and motionless. She was not breathing and the hair on the back of her neck stood up. She had spontaneous goose-bumps and her hair all over her body stood up as she knew things were not good. It was a really gripping fear. This participant could barely move from her fear. Everything inside her perceived awareness screamed against her moving herself in any way.

She attempted to talk to those shadow figures and tell them to go away, an approach that has worked for other cases in the past but was not successful with her. She would demand that they leave her, but they would still remain with her.

However, to protect her at times other than her meditating and self-hypnosis, a voice spontaneously appeared that would call her name and provide her with beautiful visions of flowering gardens and dream catchers. She thought that perhaps the voice spontaneously appeared because her apparitions became too emotionally overwhelming. On one occasion, she was almost going to hurt herself but dropped the knife when she heard the familiar woman's voice say, "No, Carey, they are not there for you." She described that voice as a grandmother's voice that was calming, soothing, and reassuring to her. This participant always thought that perhaps one of her many grandmothers was looking after her or that a spiritual guide that came to her assistance when she was weak or fearful and about to give in.

She thinks that this female voice was spiritually bonded to her as an ancestor, and would separate her from her visions when she was in real danger of losing herself in the experience. This participant believed that her ancestors had greater power and influence when compared to human beings and these shadow figures. This voice appeared when she was most terrified, often spontaneously and unexpectedly. This spontaneous voice gave her the feeling that she was not alone and an external influence was with her. It was as if someone was showing her that her family still was looking after her. She could then overcome this problem and had an ally.

She wished she had these tools of self-hypnosis to deal with the shadow figures earlier in her life. She wished someone had validated that she was having experiences with those shadow figures from which she vainly endeavored to free herself. This participant simply meditated and creatively imagined surrounding herself in white light. During her meditating, she always perceived that white light as an impenetrable armor formed by the horn of a unicorn for protection against anything that was harmful to her. She would imagine she lay inside that horn that covered over her head. She would just start at the bottom of her physical body and she would see this white light all around her. She would enter that creatively imagined horn and she would start at the bottom of her body and just cover herself all the way up and over her head. When she put the horn on over her whole body, the blacker-than-black shadow figures would slowly just dissipate or just fade away. As one shadow figure appeared, a group of wolves appeared banding together to drive the shadow figure away. For this participant, to put herself in a space where she could create white light was difficult when she was scared and gripped with fear. So every night this participant would imagine white light before she would get into her bed. She would start meditating on seeing a shield of rainbow colors protecting her and angels or wolves guarding her from the black shadow figures.

While in a self-hypnotic awareness, she would image the smoke of sage billowing all around her in a protective way like a cloud. The sage didn't remove the shadow figures, but decreased the intensity of these figures and kept them at bay. Next she put up mirrors, which did help to remove the figures on occasion, but they would eventually return later. She managed sending love and white or pink light to the figures, no thoughts just images and feelings. She would see her ancestors all around her. As a result of these exercises, her shadow figures disappeared within a month. The client has been free of these figures and all the cognitive, emotional, and behavioral side effects that came with them for seven years now. She continues to periodically practice these exercises as a preventative measure.

So as we struggle to develop a sense of ourselves in a sometimes glorious and sometimes frightening Universe, parts of us die and other parts are expanded and develop as we move into spiritual awareness and shed the cloud of illusions and false beliefs from our past and present. With this enhanced differentiation, we develop a more adaptable and flexible way of interacting with others and perceiving our world.

PERCEPTUAL POINTS

- Perceptual hypnosis helps you perceive more accurately.
- Dehypnotizing yourself is a transition that removes some of your limitations while expanding your Universe, awakening diverse perceptual possibilities, creating new positive experiences that were not possible before and broadening and deepening your connections with others.
- Perceiving more accurately can cause drastic and dramatic changes in the boundaries of your everyday life.
- New possibilities destroy old outdated beliefs that restrict your field of awareness.

PERCEPTUAL EXERCISE

Pick something that you would like to accomplish but have been fearful of achieving. It may be as simple as asking someone out on a date, trying a new food, or speaking in front of others. It may be as difficult as living alone, moving to a new geographical area away from family and friends, or starting your own business or a new career.

One possibility would be meeting someone from a different religious background or culture. You may find out that the negative characteristics that you were told these individuals possessed were not present. Rather, you might find within the person the same positive qualities you aspire to yourself. At first you might be on guard, fearful of harm, or distrustful, which later gives way to a connection and common ground, expanding your Universe to become more diverse through a new positive experience of the world.

Where else can you stretch your limits? What would it be like to heal yourself from physical illnesses? How about the experience of meeting an alien from another planet? Or to find yourself speaking to someone who holds views of the world different from your own? What would happen if you found out that death wasn't the end of your existence?

Write down spiritual, emotional, mental, and physical aspects of a fear. Notice how you experience these aspects as you approach your goal. Now, as you achieve this goal, observe and journal how these aspects change within you.

Facing your fear in this way is a mini-version of the dark night of the soul, as negative experiences and distorted perceptions flood your awareness, only to be released as you expand your sense of self and Universe with diverse possibilities and positive experiences.

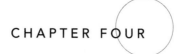

CHAPTER FOUR

PERCEPTUAL HYPNOSIS: CLEARING A PATH FOR TRUTH

Truth abhors the work of injustice, and injustice hates all the ways of truth.[40]

—*Dr. Geza Vermes*

UNDERSTANDING OF HYPNOSIS

The process of hypnosis has been viewed in different ways at different times throughout history. Each person attempts to find and explain the fundamental aspects of our consciousness or awareness manifesting themselves during hypnosis from their point of view within a certain cultural context. Mesmerism was the earliest form of hypnosis that was documented in a scholarly way. Dr. Friedrich Anton Mesmer, born in Switzerland in 1734, has been called the father of hypnosis. His dissertation at the University of Vienna asserted that the process of hypnosis utilized an invisible fluid that existed throughout the Universe. According to Mesmer, this energy was in all things.

James Braid, a medical doctor born in Kinross, Scotland, in 1795, originally coined the word "hypnosis" after the Greek god of sleep, Hypno. He later thought hypnosis would be better understood as monoideaism, or total concentration on one thought or idea. In my experience, Braid's intensely focused concentration usually involves much more, such as bodily, emotional, and mental aspects all coming together in the manifestation of one idea. The result is an expansion of your perceptual awareness.

Politicians, religious leaders, family members, advertisers, salesmen, and many other marketing professionals seek to use scientific knowledge to influence individuals like us. The best defense against this encroachment is learning and experiencing the perceptual process of hypnosis. Perceptual hypnosis shows you how to differentiate some of the multidimensional and limitless aspects of the mind in a way that enhances your life experiences. Currently, psychology attempts to compare and compete with biological sciences by placing most of its emphasis on influencing and controlling through examining thought and behavioral processes. Yet understanding of hypnosis is much more comprehensive than just a reduction to aspects of thought and behavior. Differentiation allows us to naturally enter the flow of our inner experiences, our stream of consciousness, rather than artificially isolate one aspect of the external manifestation of this stream, like snipping a weed but leaving the root. Perceptual hypnosis focuses on personal meanings, internal images, and emotions that remain invisible and immeasurable to others—quite different from concrete thoughts and behaviors, even with their multiple meanings. While members of the profession seek techniques to apply universally, they must not forget to respect individuality during the process of hypnosis so as to prevent harm through generalizations of treatment. The individual is truly the only one who can determine the full meaning of his or her experience. After all, who else would know an individual's lifetime history or the context of the person's current life experience best? A wise supervisor once stated: "We are not here to change people's reality; some fears must be respected." He then reported a story of a woman who feared going into elevators and was cured of her fear by a well-meaning behavioral therapist. She then died in an elevator crash several years later. Perhaps it would have been better to focus on enhancing her intuitive abilities, rather than blindly removing a fear.

WHAT PERCEPTUAL HYPNOSIS REVEALS

During the process of hypnosis, while the physical body relaxes, the conscious mind becomes a silent observer of a greater process within. During hypnotic experience, you are able to perceive aspects of the Universe that are not part of clear awareness in everyday life. Yet these aspects may be continually exerting an influence. Some aspects of the Universe remain in low levels of awareness, yet still affect you. That is, the Universe consists of that which you are aware of, that which you create, and that which exists without your conscious awareness of its existence. The Universe includes both publicly viewed (external and observable) and privately viewed (internal and unobservable) experience without placing a value judgment on whether one or the other is more relevant. During hypnotic experience, you are able to concentrate fully on any aspect of the Universe that you choose to understand more fully, either internal or external, or a merging of the two.

Consciousness during dehypnosis involves shifting fields of perceptual awareness. Your shifting fields determine how you creatively experience your personal world as related to the actual Universe at any moment. Thinking of Grandma's apple pie and her house takes you away from the boring drive to school. An intense focusing on the Sunday afternoon football game takes some away from all their concerns about bills, household duties, and family responsibilities. It is as if you create different fields of experience. This altering of consciousness happens in everyday life; for example, you may simultaneously perceive your significant other's anger at a distance while feeling the warmth of the beach sand on your feet. Many of my clients report not being aware of their physical bodies during hypnosis, but they are simultaneously very aware of other aspects of their experience. You may perceive various aspects of the Universe at different levels of awareness. Yet all these aspects nevertheless affect you.

Perceptual hypnosis is a spiritual phenomenon that involves accessing the very core of your being. It is more than psychological and requires a greater understanding and awareness than you might be able to grasp on your own with your conscious mind or ego. A kaleidoscopic formation taken from limitless internal and external aspects of your personal world emerges and becomes differentiated into a whole perceptual fabric at any particular moment. Hypnotic trance may be understood as those experiences that are an outcome of your altered perceptual awareness, your individual personal history, and a present yearning to maximize your potential.

When enough of your past perceptions are joined together in a present moment, a new field or gestalt of experience is created that alters your awareness back to a particular moment in time. Thus your physical body and your mind both truly perceive in a holistic manner, rather than in an "either/or" way of seeing only separate realities. Just a few aspects of a past experience may bring back the whole experience. We do not naturally experience our past or present in a detached manner. This is why some people cannot even talk about their anxiety without it creating a panic attack, and some people cry when they remember the death of a family member. Furthermore, to acknowledge many healthy and stable individuals' reports, another aspect of this kaleidoscopic experience is a perceptual awareness of a person's soul, evidenced through psychic phenomena and paranormal experiences. To holistically understand perceptual awareness, you must incorporate spiritual aspects of being human in the Universe. The truth lies in the merging of the opposites, rather than in their separation. The process of perceptual hypnosis integrates the physical and the metaphysical.

You can only grasp what you have previously perceived in the Universe—unless you learn to alter your perceptual awareness. In other words, you usually only see what you were trained to perceive and miss that which is new or different from what you are accustomed to experiencing. It is a moment of sadness when a child learns that an adult can lie or mislead them either intentionally or unconsciously, similar to Simba being lied to by Scar about his father's death. Past experience affects your ability to differentiate within the Universe, and how you see things affects how your children perceive things, as we take on what we see every day. One of my clients had a father who often would get upset when household items would break down and cost extra money to fix. When the client went out on his own, he began to also get upset when something broke down. He didn't like experiencing his father's anger, which he thought was unnecessary, as items do eventually wear out. But my client was getting just as angry as his father had in the past. Yet, it does my client little good and doesn't really fix the situation. My client's awareness allowed him to change his inner experiences, which caused the anger to begin with, so he could deal with these situations in a more adaptable fashion. He also noticed that he had a cell phone with bad reception at his home, and he infrequently would talk to his father, who would accuse him of hanging up on him when the cell signal was lost. His father often hung up on others when he didn't like the topics of conversation. These are examples of how past experiences can damage our current views. Normally you receive these suggestions in your everyday life and convert these suggestions into what you believe to be your own thoughts and actions.

I was at a party in college once where someone ordered an anchovy pizza and everyone else said things like "Yuck . . . anchovies are gross." I chose to ask a number of these people why anchovies were gross, and they told me they never had them. They had just *heard* they were gross. I went and asked if I could try a piece of anchovy pizza, and I didn't find it that bad at all. In fact, I rather liked it. This story illustrates how we sometimes take on others' beliefs about things that aren't even true without any personal experience. In addition, as memory fades with the passage of time, your own inner perceptions, such as imaginings, distorted misperceptions, and suggestions from others, may cause differences between your remembered past and what actually happened. A friend of mine had forgotten that he had put himself in harm's way one evening when he was younger, defending his brother, who was on drugs. He had, through the years, blamed his father for his difficulty with his brother. Through hypnosis he remembered having made a conscious choice with full knowledge of the possible consequences to help his brother and couldn't blame anyone but himself for his actions.

Consider how hypnosis and memory demonstrate a natural process of altering your perceptual awareness. Many people seek hypnosis to remember events from their early lives. Forgetting can be thought of as being perceptually unaware of what is happening. Forgetting and remembering are simply the everyday processes of moving perceptions into lower or higher levels of awareness. By putting an event into a low level of awareness, you put it out of your mind, so it becomes "forgotten." The process of moving experiences into a lower level of awareness is not any different from what happens when you are driving down a road and inadvertently pass the street you intended to turn onto (which was at a lower level of awareness) because you were engrossed in something else (other thoughts in a higher level of awareness). You move thoughts to different levels of awareness the same way when you turn onto the wrong street because of an old habit of driving that road to a frequent destination. The same way that driving becomes automatic in that situation, hypnosis becomes automatic as you regularly practice techniques and procedures to achieve hypnotic awareness. You may become more aware of what is influencing you in everyday life as your concentrated attention during hypnosis allows you to block out irrelevant information that is normally distracting your awareness.

HYPNOSIS AND MEMORY

When approaching the possibility of changing your consciousness or behavior, an awareness of the role memory plays within you is key. Everything you have ever learned or experienced is stored somewhere in your mind. Changes in the meaning of past events enable you to think, feel, and behave differently.

Memory is simply the storing of your perceptual experiences of your past within parts of your personal world. Not surprisingly, your present differentiations are often based on past perceptions. Dr. William Penfield, a medical doctor, demonstrated the vividness of memories when he stimulated specific areas of the brain with electrically charged needles. His patients recalled experiences as if these events were happening right before their eyes and not in the past! Penfield explained this phenomenon as ". . . a record that has not faded but seems to remain as vivid as when the record was made."[41] Experiences that you have during hypnosis are most likely carried within you in the very same way. You might retrieve or recall such experiences more easily through an understanding of perceptual awareness because they remain at low levels of awareness. In addition, your conscious mind interferes with attempts at actively perceiving memories that are stored at low levels of awareness.

In the field, there are those psychologists who believe that memory is not a literal recording but more or less an ever-changing and evolving process. In this view, your memory is continuously altered with the passage of time. Through a process of rehearsal, or recalling your past and playing memories back again and again, alterations occur each time until the original events may have little in common with your current memories of them. Images, daydreams, and for that matter television shows, commercials, video games, and virtual reality are internally recorded and also have an influence on experiences you have in the world and store as memories. At any given moment in time, when you remember, you re-experience what you have read, what you have heard about others' experiences, and even relive your dreams as immediate and real—just as immediate and as real at that moment, as when they originally occurred. As a result, you could even be unable to distinguish fact from fiction.

Perceptual hypnosis can be helpful in distinguishing what is real from what you falsely perceive in your world. Your conscious mind operating at higher levels of awareness is constantly bombarded with a great variety of daily experiences and has understandable difficulty sorting and retaining them. In fact, at lower levels of awareness, your unconscious mind is a more accurate perceiver and in tune with what really happened in the past. At some level, perhaps unconsciously (including aspects of your subconscious and spirit/soul), you may perceive the truth of a situation but have to sift through interferences from your conscious mind, with its ego distortions and deceptive beliefs—often created to defend the self against negative experiences caused by traumas, other people, and false learning—that in a way function as negative self-hypnosis. Numerous authors have provided case studies and research that validate recall of memories after accessing lower levels of awareness through hypnosis.

To accurately recall past experience during hypnosis, you have to reorganize your current perceived Universe, bringing enough aspects of it from the past into the present. At a moment in time when past emotions, images, bodily feelings, and memories of significant others are brought from lower levels into higher levels of awareness, it is possible to relive or recall an event as if it just occurred.

The sixty-seven-year-old woman who had "forgotten" her experience at Auschwitz was able to re-create the experience by bringing into higher level of awareness enough details (sounds, smells, images of faces) reminiscent of her original experience. Although this explanation may sound rather simple, unless you are aware of how your perceptual field alters your awareness, you have no way of comprehending such occurrences. Once the woman remembered it, it became clear that the event had been much more than a relatively minor incident. As a kaleidoscope has to be rearranged to visualize something perceived earlier, people need to bring enough differentiations of past experience into higher levels of awareness to recall past moments accurately. Failure to bring enough details into higher levels of awareness may result in an inability to bring past experiences into differentiation.

When working in the disaster area following hurricane Katrina in New Orleans, well-meaning adults decided to bring pet dogs to children's activities in an effort to comfort them. Sadly, when some of these children learned about this upcoming project, several re-experienced the deaths of their own pets during the flooding and were unable to attend the event. Because of their personal meanings, the children did not perceive the "therapeutic" pets as comforting.

There may also be a point when you have only partially re-created a past experience, causing a mix of both past and present perceptions. You must be patient, as moving backward or forward in time with hypnosis may take practice, and some mixture of past and present experience can occur in this process, leading, initially, to incorrect memories. You might need to undo the distorting effects of intervening experience. Any regression experience (going back into the past) can be influenced by your history since the original event. However, this does not mean that you can never accurately recall the past. You just need to be in the right level of experience to accurately recall past events. In addition, just as a joke sometimes hides a truth, there can be some symbolic truth in false memories, because you rearrange your memories to maintain and enhance your adequacy in the present moment.

A client of mine came to an understanding that as a sibling, she placed in ground the physical or sexual abuse of her sister by one of their parents during their childhood. The client hid this information by "conveniently" forgetting that her brother protected her from physical and sexual abuse. By "forgetting," she hid the fact that she sided with the abusive parent to avoid the threat of danger or sexual abuse to herself that she perceived at the time. Such post-processing of the event in the mind creates a false memory of the past. The real struggle is not to prove the self-evident—that all people might falsely recall the past—but, instead, to examine the essential aspects of past experiences after they are recalled more accurately at a later time. In this way, as the differentiation becomes clearer, people can improve their functioning and potential as human beings, rather than feeling forced to perceive themselves as helpless and unreliable victims whose memories have deteriorated over time.

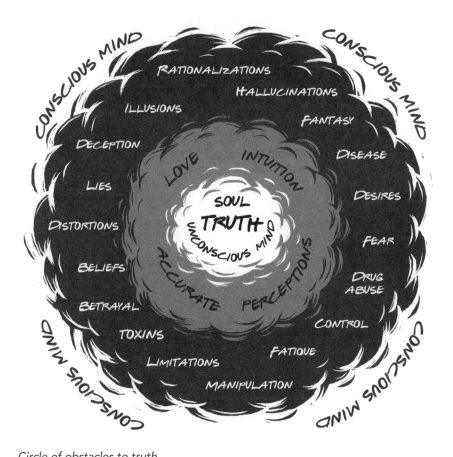

Circle of obstacles to truth.

Unfortunately, the more rigid and inflexible the person's ability to differentiate, the more likely the person will have difficulty perceiving the world accurately at any moment in time. Whenever possible, memories gathered in hypnosis should be validated with evidence from the external physical world.

My first exposure to hypnosis was a classroom demonstration conducted by a former Washington, DC, investigator, William MacDonald. He hypnotized a female student, who became unable to recall the number seven when counting from one to ten, forward or backward. During hypnosis, this woman had moved the perceptual awareness of the number seven into lower levels of her perceived Universe. She became so fully involved in the moment that she simply responded as if this hypnotist's words were true, and she let any aspects of critical thinking fade into lower levels of awareness.

On another occasion, an elderly man approached me requesting, "Hypnotize me to [help me] forget some events that took place between my wife and me." Even if hypnosis succeeded in removing the events involved from the man's conscious mind, memories of them would always be stored at some level of this individual's awareness.

During some altered levels of awareness or through suggestion by your hypnotist, you may spontaneously forget what has been occurring in a hypnotic session. In this way, memories can be remembered and forgotten, although they remain internally stored at some level of awareness, waiting to be released. Ironically, some wish to remember what they have forgotten, while others wish to forget what they remember. Although you (or any client) might distort memories under certain circumstances, these distortions have the potential to be overcome, leaving you accurately perceiving the original event.

Hypnosis has been utilized to recall childhood memories. In one case, a client remembered the circumstances and events surrounding the stealing of her family car when she was ten years old. When used to remember events earlier in your life, hypnosis is commonly called *age regression*. Age regression helps the client remember the perceptions and meanings differentiated through past events that have an effect on their present behaviors and thoughts. In another case, a young male client, who was in the habit of taking off all his jewelry before going to bed, had forgotten where he was all weekend due to a drinking spree, yet through hypnosis he was able to retrace his steps and recover his jewelry.

Hypnosis has also been utilized to recall other repressed experiences such as abuse, rape, and traumatic crimes, memories of which may occur days or weeks, even years later. In these instances, hypnosis assists you in returning to the organization of the perceived Universe that existed when the event first occurred. This same returning to an earlier organization of the Universe also happens when a posthypnotic suggestion is made to the client to be performed at some time after the hypnotic experience ends. A posthypnotic suggestion may be carried out at a later point, or when a prior hypnosis session is remembered during a new one. One spiritual goal hypnosis can address is to create personal suggestions and use them to remove outdated self-imposed posthypnotic suggestions from your experiences, your world, and from external sources, such as people you have encountered in the past.

THE THREE LEVELS OF PERCEPTUAL AWARENESS

Understanding how your perceptual awareness works is necessary to develop hypnotic abilities and skills to further enhance spiritual experiences. Perception is any differentiation an individual makes whether it is connected to an observable stimulus or not. Perception or differentiation is the source of limitless kaleidoscopic formations of merging exterior and interior experiences that include aspects of your physical senses, like touch and taste, mental images, as well as your bodily awareness, thoughts, psychic energy, and emotions. Through hypnosis, your mind, body, and spirit can work together.

One way to expand your perceptual awareness during hypnosis is to view your awareness as having three aspects:

1. A higher self
2. A conscious mind
3. A subconscious mind

A higher self is that part of your awareness that may be termed your soul. You might envision your higher self as like a guard protecting and watching over you and knowing what to let in and what to keep out. It is that part of you that knows everything and that some say can differentiate much more than can your conscious mind. People who have had near-death and out-of-body experiences explain that there is a part of their awareness that perceived everything around them during these episodes. There seems to be a lack of negative emotions such as fear, anxiety, and worry in this mode of awareness. A higher self is that part of a mother's awareness that allows her to know intuitively when her child at a distance is in distress. Some believe this self knows everything, even when your ego fails to perceive or grasp such aspects. It is the part of your awareness or mind least understood and most understudied. It is usually relegated to religion and spirituality and is mostly immeasurable. Spiritual leaders often suppress its examination, rather explaining it away in terms that describe the conscious mind rather than the higher self.

A conscious mind is that part of your self-definition that includes all the past experiences and learning you have received since birth. Your conscious mind is the part that is taught and learns from your parents, peers, schools, and culture. It is the part most studied by psychology and sociology. The conscious mind focuses on our bodies and our physical world. You are more aware of the developmental process related to this part of consciousness than you are of the other two aspects of the mind that remain less understood, partly because they are less examinable.

The subconscious mind is that aspect of you that absorbs suggestions or experience in daily living without judgment and rather concretely or literally. It can be thought of as having the mentality of a six- or eight-year-old child who doesn't know right from wrong. The subconscious mind can't reason; it doesn't know what is good or what is bad, all it knows is what it has learned. The subconscious mind recalls memories as thoughts, images, or objects. These literal learning-from-everyday-life experiences are even more potent when strong emotions are stirred up in association with them. The subconscious simply carries out desired suggestions when they are perceived as maintaining or enhancing a person's potential.

You can think of your subconscious mind as a naïve child who takes things literally and sometimes misunderstands situations and learning. What follows is an illustrative example of how your subconscious mind might interpret a situation. I conducted play therapy with an eight-year-old girl who came from a very unhappy family situation and often remained unnoticed and unacknowledged in her day-to-day life. She became upset when I walked her out to the parking lot after my last appointment and her older brother was late to pick her up. She only lived up the street, so I said, "Don't worry, the worst that can happen is that I'll take you home." My intention was to drive her to her home, but she interpreted my statement as meaning that I was going to rescue her from her unhappy circumstances and take her to my home. Her interpretation shows exactly how the subconscious mind works, potentially misperceiving suggestions from personal life experiences and developing new creative or destructive patterns. This consciousness is the part of the mind most targeted by external influences (advertising and marketing, politics, media, and economic leaders) to mold and shape your behavior while you remain unaware of the underlying motives affecting you so strongly.

Everything that happens during hypnosis also happens in everyday life experiences. For instance, some spiritual people have spoken of simultaneously experiencing two levels of communication with another person: an outside verbal and an inside thought level, effectively having two conversations with that person at the same time. For example, a research subject reported hearing his professor lecturing while he heard his own dog yelp in his mind as he sat in the classroom. He next heard his own mind saying his dog's name, and then heard his professor's voice in his mind say, "That's not my dog," as if the professor knew the student had just heard his dog yelp. This happened while his professor continued to lecture to the class. When the young man went home, he found his dog had chewed a soda can and had cut his mouth. Later, he found out that his professor also had a dog. The events in a story like this one may be attributed to psychic abilities, coincidence, or divine powers. If you fear or don't understand something, you suppress it; if it is in line with your beliefs, then you might attribute it to a divine power. One response might be the fact that the professor had a dog isn't noteworthy, since so many people do. However, for this individual it was very scary and personal to him that voices in his head had provided him with information that later proved correct that he couldn't possibly know at the time. If his experience was perceived accurately, it suggests a dissolving of the boundaries of time and distance in perception.

Perceptual awareness involves exploring boundless possibilities in relationship to the self. By narrowing perceptions, people often create their own limitations. One of the greatest philosophical arguments of all times has to do with the essence of perceptual awareness: what really does and does not exist in the Universe? Some need to perceive something to believe it, while others believe without perceiving.

ORGANIZING AN INDIVIDUAL PERCEIVED UNIVERSE

For individuals, the present organization of their perceived Universes—those aspects of their personal worlds that are in higher levels of conscious awareness as well as aspects that remain at low levels of awareness—constitute their current reality. Your present need is to fulfill and enhance, to the best of your ability, all aspects of your life. Thus, differentiation and this need to maximize potential determine what you perceive, and that is how you create a personal perceived Universe.

Perceptual theory has defined a human being's basic need as a "need for adequacy" or maintenance and enhancement of the self, an active process. In the literature the process is described as:

> that biologically grounded force in each of us by which we are continually seeking to make ourselves ever more adequate to cope with life. Whether we seek to maintain ourselves as we are or enhance ourselves against the exigencies of the future, we are always seeking to be the most adequate persons we can be.[42]

Perceptual awareness includes all the ways that you become aware of fulfilling your needs in the Universe, both visible and invisible. Perceptual awareness also unites one moment with the next moment and allows you to recognize meaning in your life. You are only aware of what exists for you in your perceived Universe. You have developed a network of perceptions from infancy, one personal experience after another, creating a personal history.

Your perceived Universe exists only as you differentiate it and only for as long as you remain unchanged. This Universe is a combination of both your individual perceived Universe, as you created it with all its distortions, and the Universe as it truly and accurately exists, differentiated or not. The more accurately we perceive the closer we come to the truth as it actually exists. For example, if there is an afterlife, it exists independently of your belief in its existence. If there is reincarnation, rebirth is not stopped by your disbelief in it. When you change a perception, it may change the totality of your perceived self and perceived Universe. The perceived Universe and the actual Universe are two different things, and the perceived Universe is more open to change since it also includes some distortions. This change can be thought of as parallel to looking through a kaleidoscope. Images viewed in a kaleidoscope are constantly merging, joining, and separating, each combination creating its own little image. A limitation to this analogy is that a kaleidoscope has few combinations compared to the myriad of possibilities, limitless in nature, for experience in the world.

CONNECT RATHER THAN PROJECT—AWAKENING FROM THE SLEEP

Historically, perceptual hypnosis maintains a phenomenological stance of setting aside biases while allowing meaning to naturally unfold in its own way and time. Phenomenology seeks the simplest and most basic understanding of experience through examining individuals' verbal descriptions of life events. Phenomenology originated in Germany and France at the turn of the last century with the works of philosophers Edmund Husserl, Martin Heidegger, and Maurice Merleau-Ponty. It seeks the essence of life and the bottom-line meaning that experience holds for each individual person.

As Dr. Clark Moustakas, a humanistic psychologist, stated: "The word 'phenomenon' comes from the Greek 'phaenesthai': to flare up, to show itself, to appear . . . Phenomena are the building blocks of human science and the basis for all knowledge."[43] Dr. Moustakas believed that experience was the foundation of scientific investigation. Dr. Ludwig Binswanger, a psychiatrist who studied under Carl Jung, defined the phenomenological approach as:

> devot[ing] itself to the phenomenal content of every verbal expression, every mode of action, every attitude, and attempts to understand it from basic modes of human existence prior to the separation of body, soul, and mind, and of consciousness and unconsciousness. . . .[44]

In this way, perceptual hypnosis differs from the many psychological theories that project meaning onto peoples' situations based on the examiner's past experiences and while ignoring the vast possibilities of diverse situations that the examiner may not have experienced. In that way, not setting aside bias in the examiner can lead clients to fear the expression of experiences being judged in a negative light in a restrictive range of possibilities, sometimes despite being well adjusted and adequately functioning in their lives.

When you are phenomenological in your view, you are able to see as much as possible of another's perceived Universe, rather than remaining rigidly in a reality outside their perceptual awareness. To see phenomenologically is to see the world through their eyes. This approach usually makes others feel safe, as they are being heard or understood and connected to by you. This is a difficult and time-consuming process at first, as a person needs to set aside past learning that could interfere with seeing something in a new way. This may sound simple but is a rather difficult process and requires unlearning some basic biases. When encountering a novel experience, we often almost instantly go to our past experiences to understand it. Sheldon B. Kopp, psychotherapist, pointed this out long ago, when speaking of a minister as a counselor:

> Like the psychiatrist, the clinical psychologist, and the psychiatric social worker, the minister must not only survive his training but also transcend it, if he is to become a responsible spiritual guide who knows what he is doing. The minister, too, must find some way to be illumined, to unlearn what he has been taught, and to learn that which cannot simply be taught.[45]

You are more helpful if you connect with others' perceptual awareness and do not project your own perceptual distortions on them. You do not connect when you project. For example, for you to receive an omen or a spiritual sign, you first have to place an individual and unique meaning on the events and occurrences that you experience. You have to choose to be open to a spiritual symbol, sign, or living being for it to become a messenger. A spiritual sign has a distinctively individual meaning. For example, I often see a fox run across the road or in the woods when someone in a position of power in my life is attempting to take unfair advantage of me. A client of mine would know a situation was okay when she would see two animals playing or walking together, such as two porcupines, which is by the way, not a very commonly viewed event in most places.

One evening in my hometown as I was struggling with a decision I had to make over working with my clients and my clinical practice, I walked across a small bridge near my office. I was halfway across this bridge, when an animal began to enter the bridge from the other side and came toward me. It was late at night, and I became wary as it was not a house cat or a domestic dog, and I could feel the movement of the bridge with each step the animal took toward me. It was a gray fox that stopped about a foot from my body for a few moments and looked directly in my eyes before moving past me. This encounter focused me and helped me make a very crucial decision in my life. I would never have had this encounter with this fox if I acted out of fear or aggression. Symbols hold both universal and uniquely individual meaning that others cannot control or determine.

Another example of a symbol may be seeing a blue bird as a sign that you have made a correct decision. In such circumstances, the internal sense of certainty is validated externally when a blue bird appears in your field of awareness and the situation turns out as intuited. A person with a spiritual background may have such a perception. If you are a less spiritual person, you may not make such connections even

Fox on the bridge.

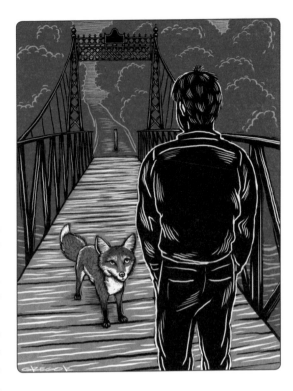

if they are present in your surroundings. On the opposite side of the view, psychotic people see such connections where there are none. An adequate personality seeks relationships and connectedness. As a result of caring about relating, an adequate personality takes personal and social responsibility, and emphasizes social justice and the welfare of others in everyday life. Dr. Buscaglia described an experiment conducted in a sociology class that relates to this tendency. The students were required to donate ten cents. Their money could go to both women and children who were dying from a disaster in India, a black student who, through family misfortune, was unable to continue his college education, or toward a Xerox machine that would allow students to make free copies. Results of a secret ballot were as follows: 85 percent went to the Xerox machine, 12 percent went to the black student, and only 3 percent went to the dying women and children![46] What do these choices say about the adequacy of the students' personalities? Only 15 percent of the students showed that they experienced a sense of relationship and connectedness with people.

I conducted an experiment with several high school classes, presenting teenage students with a scene in a public park: A teenager had a sandwich he was about to eat when an elderly woman walked by him, picked up a peanut off the ground, and ate it. When asked what they would do in this situation, seventy students said they would not assist the old woman, explaining that authority figures told them not to talk to strangers. Ten students said they would give their sandwiches to this old woman. Only two female students stated that they would keep half of their sandwich and give the other half to her. This result shows how dehumanizing perceptions of others can be, how people can view other people from different walks of life as objects separate from themselves. Such separation is an enemy of spirituality, as the Universe is, in reality, interconnected and joined.

You cannot escape the fact that you are always in relationship with the Universe around you. As you attempt to look accurately at the Universe with impartial eyes, without prejudice or bias, you do so while still being a part of it. As you are looking at some aspect of your perceived Universe, it is important to realize that you are a part of the Universe through your experience. Your link with nature is evidenced by the fact that you need plant life for the oxygen you breathe. You are of nature and intimately in relationship with nature in a shared space with the whole of the Universe.

Doreen, an ex-girlfriend of mine, told me that it made her sad when she went to a beach and watched everybody leaving litter around and thought about how this is happening all over the Earth. She was capable of perceiving the planet as a living and essential contributor to human survival and well-being. If the planet dies, so will all human beings!

In direct contrast to this woman's perception of the world, an acquaintance of mine confessed that after changing the oil for his truck, he would secretly discard the old oil anywhere he could without any concern for the environment. His reasoning: to save a few dollars at the waste disposal site. Along these lines, there are many crimes against humanity grounded in economic justifications. Some people intentionally make equipment and machinery that will become obsolete, rather than last a lifetime. Some unethical landlords fail to properly insulate tenants' housing to save a few dollars for themselves, forcing their tenants to consume more fuel and the community to ultimately deal with more damage to the environment. When people misperceive others and nature as objects separate from themselves, it leads to many atrocities, including the poisoning of essential elements of human existence (such as air and water). Conversely, persons who experience true love or a concept of oneness realize their relationship with the Universe and perceive an interlocking unity of all things. Thus, how persons see themselves determines how they act toward others and respond to the Universe.

PERCEPTUAL POINTS

- Through differentiation, perceptual hypnosis helps us create different fields of experience.
- Everything that happens during hypnosis also happens in everyday life experiences.
- The Universe is a combination of both your individual perceived Universe, as you created it with all its distortions, and the Universe as it truly and accurately exists, differentiated or not.

EXERCISE 1

One way to expand your perceptual awareness in hypnosis is to view your awareness as having three levels during hypnosis: a higher self, a conscious mind, and a subconscious mind. Concentrate on getting in touch with these three parts of your mind by:

Using your creative imagination to visualize yourself in a very relaxing situation. Imagine a time when you were really relaxed. Maybe you were sun tanning, lying on the grass looking up at the clouds, fishing from a canoe, or just relaxing in your favorite chair on a beautiful day on the porch of your favorite place while feeling a gentle breeze. Your mind was free of any troubles or worries. Your body just let go of any tension or stress and you were slowly awakening the higher self and your own intuitive knowledge. Imagine that your conscious mind has agreed to open that door to greater awareness and your subconscious mind has pictures of you changing and expanding into something greater. The thoughts slowly disappear as you are in the moment now. Let that greater part of you come forward. Imagine that there is no time or space, and you can go anywhere, be anywhere, in an instant. Picture yourself looking down at the earth from above the sky, seeing all around you, 360 degrees, or just seeing a deer drinking water at a lake far beyond your physical eye's capabilities at this moment.

Observing your awareness passively in the present moment. What are you perceiving at the moment? Just let yourself go; just let your self be still. After this experience try to describe it in words and write it down.

Using your imagination and observing your own awareness will allow these aspects of yourself to unfold. You will naturally expand your awareness over time.

EXERCISE 2

Attempt a phenomenological experiment by really listening to what another person is saying. Tell the person what you think you heard or ask him/her to further explain things if you don't understand the words. This action will help increase your intimacy in close relationships and help you avoid projecting yourself on others, improving your relationships overall. Pay attention to your use of judgmental words like "good, bad, unhealthy, and positive," and ask questions.

EXERCISE 3

List all the connections you have in your life that are essential for your daily living. For example, physically you need plants in order to breathe. You need someone who cares about you in order to share your feelings. What spiritual connections do you have with the Universe? Then go into self-hypnosis as we described earlier (and at the end of the book), and explore your connections.

HYPNOTIC KNOWLEDGE AS PROTECTION

What we consider supernatural becomes natural, while that which we have always seen as so natural reveals how wondrously supernatural it is.[47]

—Dr. Frederick Franck

Perceptual hypnosis offers a form of psychological immunization or vaccination for your mind, a preventive measure for your soul, much like vitamins taken for the physical body. In today's society there are numerous influences affecting each individual, and the only danger of hypnosis is that the uninitiated are unaware of how its principles are encountered in everyday life. You can be in danger when someone says something to you and you act on it without even realizing the influence that statement exerted on you. Often you do not even know if such a statement is accurately representing the Universe.

Here's an everyday example of how we can become influenced without even knowing our behavior is being shaped: A roommate of mine went out sledding in the snow with his girlfriend and her son. He saw my gloves lying around and borrowed them. He asked me later when he was finished if those were my gloves. When I told him they were, he went on to tell me in detail about how much fun he had had in the snow and how I should go sledding. He stated: "You need to go buy yourself a hat, a scarf, and some gloves." I did not take to his suggestion. After I waited a few hours to see if he would return them, I finally asked for my gloves back.

One reason awareness of hypnotic principles of communication is necessary is to reduce negative external and internal influences that may undermine the expression of your potential in life or your relationships. Ultimately the use of perceptual hypnosis is to develop these characteristics of the adequate personality. Spiritual individuals or healers perceive another's needs as relevant and important in and of themselves, regardless of any "payoff" they themselves might receive. How persons treat others reveals how they truly perceive them. Through observing as a third party the interactions between others, you can spot true genuineness about, or lack of concern for, a sense of community and the welfare of other human beings. An example of such identification with others is found in a story that occurred during World War II. During the Germany occupation, King Christian of Denmark stood up as a true leader of his people when the Germans mandated that all Jews from Denmark wear yellow stars so that they could be easily identified and transported to concentration camps. To express his opposition to the German mandate and protect his country men and women, King Christian put a yellow star on his own clothes, and most of the people of Denmark followed suit, preventing the Germans from identifying who was or was not a Jew! This move by the king was the act of an adequate personality, putting his peoples' welfare before his own.[48] King Christian demonstrated the characteristics of an adequate personality as described in *Perceptual Psychology* by Drs. Combs, Richards and Richards.[49] A person or leader with an adequate personality would have these traits:

- An open and flexible perceived Universe
- An ability to identify with others
- Positive experiences in his or her world
- A rich diversity of personal meanings and perceptions of the world

A person of this type would be better able to protect freedom of thought and self-empowerment and would not be interested in controlling or manipulating others. The relationship style would be direct and honest.

King Christian put himself at risk for his people, while Hitler put his people at risk for himself. Similarly, Simba in *The Lion King* put himself at risk by returning to defend his pride from Scar, who had used the pride for his own advantage and had destroyed the land while pursuing his own need for power. King Christian and Simba demonstrate the qualities of the adequate personality, just as King Solomon did in ancient times, when he was able to determine the true mother of a child. When two women came forward claiming to be the child's mother, King Solomon determined who was the true mother by ordering the child to be cut in half and for each mother to be given a half. The true mother sacrificed herself and insisted the false mother be given the child. King Solomon, whose perceived Universe encompassed diverse perceptual possibilities, was able to differentiate or identify the true mother and return the child to her. Without accurately perceiving we cannot act in our own best interests and may be led astray like lemmings over a cliff. Simba did not accurately perceive the cause of his father's death until the end of the movie, when he began to see how his Uncle Scar was endangering the pride. He then uncovered Scar's lies, which he had taken as truth up until that point.

All communication is perceptually hypnotic in its essence. Are you aware of the messages coming your way? Being aware of body language, gestures, and expressions between yourself and others in your life can enable you to understand your relationships more deeply. This is an example of sharing each other's perceived Universe. The ability to perceive emotions in others and to discern how others are feeling is sometimes described as intuition. It can also be described as unconsciously perceiving others at low levels of awareness. You may also use other terms that show the difficulty of classifying such energy or feelings. For such an exchange to occur between them, individuals share some aspects of each other's perceived Universe. Some have even referred to this phenomenon as psychic energy, which science finds hard to describe or define.

SEEING THROUGH THE LIES AND ILLUSIONS

A deep search of your heart and soul will make you aware of some aspect of yourself that needs to grow and develop. Growth and development of the self shouldn't really stop until you die (and maybe it won't end then either!). Some of you are even reaching for peak experiences that will allow you to transform yourselves—reorganize the perceived self—to see the world in an entirely new way. Hopefully, those of you seeking self-actualization will come across the right sort of experiences and people to help you fulfill your potential. Of course, if you want to reach past perceived limitations, you need only shatter false realities; you then perceive things more accurately! For example, when Roger Bannister became the first runner to break the four-minute mile in 1954, he broke both physiological and psychological barriers, and soon, other runners around the world were running a mile in under four minutes.

People often seek facts to support their view of their perceived Universe rather than trying to accurately or more objectively perceive the Universe. Many individuals jump to conclusions quickly without the proper information or experience to truly judge or even comprehend the significance of many occurrences in their everyday lives. People often assert their personal truth as the Truth. They seek friends who validate their reality and information that supports the beliefs that sustain their lifestyles.

Not surprisingly, there is no instrument that can measure human experience better than your own inner self. When you accept something at face value and do not check out its validity, it is as if you are creating a "suggestion" to yourself to perceive the world in a particular way. For example, such statements as "you're too young to own a house" or "you're too old to have a family" become excuses to not take action, rather than being factual. These statements demonstrate everyday hypnosis is imposed on you by others to conform to their reality. Your greatest task is to seek knowledge that leads to uncovering the wisdom of universal truths, rather than reiterating group or individual biases.

Perceptual theory shows you how social interaction with other people and their alternative perceptions can affect you. Influences from others and their past experiences can either restrict or expand your spiritual development as they attempt to pass their perceptual awareness on to you. You either voluntarily or involuntarily lose or gain the power to perceive new possibilities in your life.

FREEDOM OF THOUGHT COMES FROM NEW DIFFERENTIATIONS

How you perceive the Universe has a major impact on how your everyday life proceeds. Your perceptual awareness is the basis for all the meaning you derive in life; your perceptions create the possibilities that lead to your reactions to everything that happens to you. Who knows your experiences better than you? Are outside influences affecting how and what you perceive? Almost everyone is hypnotized without being aware of this at some point or another. Any time you take on a fact as true, when it is not, and act as if it is real, you have been hypnotized by someone else. This is why I call what I do *dehypnotizing*. I'm allowing you to see reality for what is truly there for you, rather than shaping the world falsely with distortions that suit you or others' limited frame of reference. These distortions are heavily connected to fears and emotions that guard against any change or new differentiations for fear of losing one's self. Some people fear that new differentiation means losing yourself, but this couldn't be further from the truth, since losing distortions through new differentiations allows you to become freer to pursue your real purpose in life and live a deeper and happier existence. Freeing you like this also takes away the power of others to manipulate and alter your perceptions for their own benefit.

As you create new ideas, perceptions, thoughts, and resulting words and behaviors, you change your life. Any time you change the focus of your attention onto your body or some aspect of your environment, you can go into a light trance. The power lies within us, not outside of us. We can alter our worlds and enhance our lives if we wish to. When I was a novice hypnotherapist, I began working out of the basement of the home I was renting. My roommate had a small dog that often barked incessantly. While hypnotizing a new client, I completely put the dog out of my awareness. However, when we were done, I found out the client was unable to get the dog's barking out of his mind. I was able to change my environment because I had learned how to unleash my potential, but he had not yet.

Such a change in differentiation is a change in our personal world. A more important idea is: Will you allow yourself to become knowingly dehypnotized, to become aware of how thoughts and perceptual awareness affect your body, emotions, mind, and spirit through new and more accurate perceptions?

SHIELDING YOURSELF FROM NEGATIVE INFLUENCE OF OTHERS

You can start with your well-meaning family and friends. So many of their words and images often slide into your mind without your taking the slightest notice! Then there are those with embedded, hidden answers in their questions. You do not have to accept these negative limiting perceptions that affect you unknowingly at multiple levels and prevent growth in your life. You can reverse these negative statements and enhance your life. "Aren't you too old to be playing softball?" For example, "I enjoy playing softball, and I have noticed how I have improved in my performance over the last month." "If you write that book, who is going to read it?" Replace this with, "My book will enhance the lives of those who are interested in similar pursuits." "Hypnosis . . . can you really control someone else's mind?" Rather, "Hypnosis helps me to take control of my own mind." The false assertions: "It will take a lifetime to pay off that debt!"; "The weather is bad; you won't be able to go to work today." The presenters of false facts: "I couldn't afford to live where you live; the cost of living is too high"; "If you stop lifting weights, you will lose the muscle in a few weeks"; "Oh, as you get older your metabolism slows, your body becomes overweight, and your body tissue begins to sag"; "When you have children, you will be as overweight as me." So many suggestions, and just how did they arise? Who first proposed such self-limiting assertions? The answer of course is that other people did. Write down some more rational open-minded thoughts and ideas that point out the reverse of such limiting suggestions. Make it a habit to become aware of these influences and stop them with counter self-suggestions.

You can learn to recognize such positive and healthy influences in the Universe and to filter out unwanted negative ones. As the great hypnotist Dr. Milton H. Erickson, MD, stated: "Usually when I talk to people, some hypnosis is involved."[50] When you accept ideas or thoughts from others without question or further investigation as to their truth or falsity, you risk accepting a false statement or a distortion of reality as a living reality in your perceived Universe. In this way, you can be hypnotized into a false reality in everyday life without even knowing there are alternatives for you.

Others' influences can also have positive effects, as they expand our awareness. For instance, you might remember a high school teacher or other adult who encouraged you in your goals and dreams. Throughout my life, my maternal grandfather, William Abel, reminded me, "Your mind can do incredible things, Fred." As thoughts and images, these influences can have a great impact on a person's life and perceptual awareness if accepted as true. Affirmative communication and positive thinking are not simply forms of suggestion to self or others. These ideas instead branch out into images, feelings, and interactions with the Universe. An everyday example of conscious expansion of our perceptions occurred for me when, after a motorcycle accident, I walked around the block while recovering and was able to walk well. To some observers, and perhaps my own observations in the past, I was able to walk normally around the block, so for them and my old self views, I had recovered nicely. However, for the next two days, I could barely walk without excruciating pain throughout my leg. When I held the idea that I felt fine, I was okay at the moment of walking. This could not automatically be generalized to a later time, however. Therefore, I became more aware of the disadvantages of suffering from physical injuries and corrected distorted perceptions of their unrealistic well-being. A spiritual example is when you begin to realize that someone can know something about you without needing to be physically present to you, such as with clairvoyance, telepathy, and remote viewing. You can panic and get paranoid or angry and feel it is not possible and you must be going crazy, or that the other person is evil. Once you grow to understand this idea, however, you can find a new faith and trust in the Universe. When something alters your perceptual awareness, it can have great and expanding side effects.

Experiencing hypnosis can make you aware that negative remarks and suggestions made by peers and persons in authority are often more in line with their personal meanings in life than with your own goals and needs. Perceptual hypnosis involves gaining self-control of your mind, rather than giving it away to outside control. One of my mentors, on hearing that my first manuscript was going to be published, smiled with his eyes gleaming and his body language expressing his sincere happiness for me. Another professor responded by stating that journal articles are just jargon the average person can't understand and that the more difficult task may be to write for diverse populations and not just for one group of readers. By not just accepting all responses at face value, I could keep control over my own mind. I could choose:

- To accept the positive support from the first professor
- To consider a new direction, as suggested by the second professor—reaching a lay audience, rather than writing only for professional journals—without abandoning my goals
- To not be discouraged by professors who made less supportive statements, whether they were intentionally trying to discourage me or not

My mentor, Dr. Anne Cohen-Richards, reassured me after my first manuscript was initially rejected, "Fred, you know Rollo May was rejected a number of times before his first book was published. This was also true of Abe Maslow's second book." Another professor said, "It's very difficult to get published; I wouldn't make that a priority." Ten published journal articles later, I pondered how people are often unaware of the ways that they are being influenced, whether positively or negatively.

Perceptual influences are even more basic than verbal suggestions, often passing through your critical faculties unnoticed. You are more often aware of your words and less often aware of the perceptions that are at their foundation. Suggestions become thought control when you accept anonymous opinions or absolute statements as truth, regardless of whether or not such conclusions are based in fact. Just like a posthypnotic suggestion (a lingering effect after the hypnotic trance is over), your everyday behavior is altered by taking on even one of these little false statements or distorted facts as incorrectly true. You might perceive a statement as a fact, or seeming fact, and as true, depending on the frame of reference utilized by the person making the assertion. Often a child accepts as true a statement made by a parent. For example, just before administering an intelligence test to a child, I overheard his mother say within hearing range of this child, "Oh, I don't think my child will be anything but average." How unfortunate for this child, who might interpret this statement as factual and never aspire to greater achievement. Often statements in conversation are not statements of fact, but statements to influence another as if they were fact.

Hypnosis is actually a means for you to learn just what and how you are affected by other people's influences, and how others' statements have an impact on you. Hypnotic experience provides a way to identify influences all around you in everyday life. At one point in my life, whenever I was out socializing, I became aware that I had never met the wrong party in a divorce, but always the party who was the victim! I must have been in all the right places at all the right times. I would guess that among the ten real estate agencies in town, each employee perceives his or her respective agency as the agency that best serves the public in that town. Clearly, by definition, only one can be the best, unless they are all tied for first place.

If you are going to take responsibility for your life, you not only need to understand how others affect you, but also need to understand how you affect the perceptions of others. Your actions and words can alter others' perceptions and personal meanings, changing the course of their lives for better or for worse. Perceptual hypnosis can allow you to break down and re-experience perceptions that are lumped together and falsely appear as one event, allowing the many different aspects of that experience to unfold. Such awareness can unleash unknown spiritual potential while increasing everyday personal control and awareness. Of course, this requires taking personal responsibility for your life and no longer playing the role of the victim of outside influences.

Talking with others can provide you with alternative perceptions of a situation, but which perception is most accurate? It is always better to seek out people who have maximized their potential in a particular area of life. Such individuals are more likely to be objective about your situation and give unbiased knowledge with your best interests in mind, rather than giving you distorted information in an attempt at fulfilling a personal need of their own or comparing your need to theirs. The less adequate people's personalities are, the less able they are to help others since their personal meanings and need to maximize potential are distorted, restricting their capacity to see alternatives in the Universe. In other words, more experiences doesn't always mean more self-knowledge, since a person might never have developed an ability to see diverse possibilities, but might instead have a tendency to use the same cookie-cutter mold for all interactions.

A scientist, a hypnotist, and a toddler are all attempting to grasp new understandings through creating and exploring experiences. They are intensely focused on higher levels of awareness. At the same time, they are moving familiar aspects of their Universes into lower levels of awareness. When children perceive a future event in their minds and later it comes true, they have no understanding of how that could have happened based on their everyday life experiences. It is something they did not expect and do not know how to explain. Later they come to learn that there are others who have had those experiences and begin to expand their consciousness. Adults who see a ball of energy bouncing around at night in the street and have no past experience to explain it, find the occurrence seems alien. They later may come to understand that it does happen to a few other people. These individuals now have an expanded consciousness not available to everyone. I assume experiences of those credited with the great scientific discoveries were similar, such as when scientists perceived the ideas that blood circulates in our bodies and that the earth revolves around the sun. It is this process of differentiating unfamiliar aspects of the Universe coupled with the process of exercising the flexibility to perceive diverse aspects of a personal world that allows persons to grow physically, emotionally, mentally, and spiritually. This ability to experiment and take risks in life allows people's perceptual potentialities to expand. All behavior is a result of what people perceive to be the best possible action that they can take at a given moment. These processes of differentiating and maintaining and maximizing potential are the keys to understanding perceptual aspects of hypnosis and to expanding perceptual awareness.

PERCEPTUAL POINTS

- Practicing perceptual hypnosis can be likened to taking an immunization or vitamins, providing protection against outside influences.
- Awareness of the ways that outside forces try to inflict suggestion on others can protect you from their influence.
- Freedom of thought that comes from new differentiations is the true power of hypnosis.

PERCEPTUAL EXERCISE

Creatively imagine something that widens or expands your perceived Universe every day. Take a risk a day to expand your whole life by experiencing more of what there is in the Universe. For example:

- Look around your room and notice everything, including what you have often ignored.
- Step outside and look for something you never noticed in your neighborhood.
- Watch what's happening in the background in a movie or on television.
- Listen to what people aren't saying, instead of what they are emphasizing in conversation.
- Notice what they are saying with the expressions of their body movements, facial expressions, the words they choose to use, and their expressions.
- Take a negative statement and explore all the possible positive aspects of this experience that you can for yourself or for another person. Try to see the statement from a different perspective.

Each night before you go to bed, or before you get up in the morning or as you awaken, try to picture in your mind a goal for the following day that will expand your perceived Universe. Make the image as clear as possible. Later write down what your mind created, paying attention to every little detail of your imagining.

Conversely, if you are overstimulated, you can narrow your perceptual field. It may seem like a small step, but changing perceptions has a way of generating transformation that may blossom into what you would like to see in your life. During each day, be aware of when and where you restrict your perceptions and narrow your perceived Universe, and plan future risks and goals based on these observations.

SELF-HYPNOSIS EXERCISE

Imagine creating a protective shield or bubble around yourself and visualize various ways of connecting to a great source of brilliant white light. Be creative and use inner self-exploration. Change the color from white to red to orange to yellow to green to blue to purple to indigo. See the various colors as layers protecting and soothing you. You can imagine protective beings like angels, your ancestors, or animals guarding you. Open up to interactions with the greater Universe.

CHAPTER SIX

DEFINITIONS OF HYPNOTIC PHENOMENA IN PERCEPTUAL THEORY

So we begin with ourselves, gaining control of our own minds, then helping others as the effective hypnotist does, to be in control of their minds.[51]

—Dr. Joel Fort

Before going any further, I'd like to define and discuss some types of hypnotic experiences that I refer to in this book. Being familiar with the particular hypnotic phenomena that typically occur prepares you to better understand the effect that hypnosis can have on your life. Remember that such phenomena are occurring every day at low levels of awareness in your own daily life, so you probably will recognize them in yourself or others. While being hypnotized by a trained professional, you can experience:

- Time distortion
- Age regression
- Pseudo-orientation in time
- Amnesia, hypermnesia, paramnesia, and crytomnesia
- Positive hallucinations
- Negative hallucinations
- Analgesia and anesthesia
- Post-hypnotic suggestion
- Catalepsy
- Subconscious manifestations
- Somnambulism

TIME DISTORTION

Time distortion is a hypnotic phenomenon related to your capacity to experience the speeding up (expansion) or slowing down (contraction) of clock time through an altering of perceptual awareness. When this occurs, your personal world is altered as you shift to higher levels of awareness in time expansion; or to lower levels of awareness in time contraction. You lose yourself in expanded awareness as time seems to speed up and your sense of yourself loses its boundaries of confinement. You mind embraces a much greater self-definition than the limitations of your physical body. You become vividly self-conscious when you return to normal reality and time slows down. You forget that human beings subjectively create their experience of time, and hypnotic perceptual awareness allows you to step out of a clock-time frame of reference long enough to acknowledge human experience outside it.

You can explore the process of differentiating or perceiving different aspects of your personal world in nonlinear experience, where time and distance are not relevant to your expanded awareness. It is as if you become a ball of energy without a body or without relationship to material things. You know mentally that you're aware, but you have no awareness of your body.

Many clients have reported such altered levels of perceptual awareness during hypnosis and that experiencing them changed the way they perceived movement and experienced time and space for a particular event, such as completing an activity in ten seconds that normally takes sixty minutes. A proper understanding of this perceptual awareness of time during hypnosis can help prolong or shorten the perception of time for your benefit in your everyday experiences. Dr. Linn F. Cooper and Dr. Milton Erickson demonstrated a perceptual technique during a hypnosis session that condensed relevant aspects of a dental assistant's problem dealing with patient blood from a significant period of time in her daily work routine to inner perceptions and images lasting only a matter of seconds. They further demonstrated that changing perceptions can alter perceived time. For example, time passed slowly and seconds seemed like minutes or hours to some clients during hypnotic experience. Drs. Cooper and Erickson stated: "Such subjects may routinely report having finished 'completed' tasks, whose seeming duration is thirty to sixty minutes, in an allotted time (A.T.) of three seconds."[52]

Thus, hypnosis can be a powerful and effective therapeutic intervention when addressing the perception of time. You can lengthen your pleasant experiences and shorten your unpleasant moments in time. Your mind naturally expands or contracts your experience of time to protect you during trauma. For example, as mentioned earlier, I remember being hurled from my motorcycle after a head-on collision with a car. I felt myself sail through the air and hit the ground as my helmet and head bounced up from the pavement. I perceived my elbow hit the side of the road, and watched my wrist bend in slow motion and shatter. This occurred in what seemed like a slowed down version of clock time but was only a matter of a few seconds. My mind protected me from the negative aspects of the trauma by slowing down my mind's perception of the event in ways we really don't even understand. When you experience trauma, your mind seems to naturally use hypnotic experience to see you through such a situation.

AGE REGRESSION

Age regression is a reorganizing of your perceived Universe and self to include past experience within a present moment in time. Psychiatrist Milton Erickson and psychologist Ernest Rossi believed that during age regression an individual moves to an earlier phase of personality development. As you move more aspects of past experience into higher levels of awareness, you begin to revivify the experience or relive it as it occurred at an earlier moment in time.

Revivification is recapturing or reliving a prior experience as if it were occurring at this moment in time, with the present fading into lower levels of awareness. During revivifying, a past moment becomes your entire perceived Universe. For example, a client might not be aware of the hypnotist or experience self as an adult; rather he perceives himself as a seven-year-old child. In this particular case, all of an individual's life experience after the age of seven is placed in lower levels of awareness, and the client becomes frozen in time.

Naturally occurring regressions happen in everyday life when you are reunited with members of your original family, or at times of stress in an intimate relationship when you revert to earlier experiences. You may be taken back in time through a smell or a taste, or an aspect of the environment that appears exactly like what you encountered in a past experience. What seems crucial for age regression to occur is that enough aspects that replicate the original experience are present to move you back into recalling or reliving past experience. Clients go through age regression when similar things happen that trigger old repressed memories or awaken potential they had forgotten. Age regression can be helpful in processing material that was too threatening at the time it occurred. Later, however, the person has grown and is more able to handle the experience in the present than they were in the past.

PSEUDO-ORIENTATION IN TIME

Pseudo-orientation in time involves the perception of a possible future event or a review of your life in the present from a point five years in the future. You might reflect on consequences and impact of making life changes, or for that matter what will happen if these changes are not made. How you perceive an aspect of your Universe at this moment in time may affect how you differentiate experiences from the past and into the future. New knowledge may expand the meaning of old experiences.

Pseudo-orientation in time allows you to change your perception of the past, present, and future, as a way to bring a more adequate understanding of it into the present. Through a change in perceptual awareness, you can create hypnotic experience that reorganizes your perceived Universe. For example, you might experience a positive interaction with others in the future that allows your present experience to draw you closer to your goals.

Using pseudo-orientation in time, you can explore a time before a traumatic or threatening experience occurred, such as the encouraging words of a grandparent before he or she died. Or you can move forward to a time when a particular experience will be resolved and no longer affecting you, such as what it is like to graduate, quit smoking, or stand up to a bully at school. You may perceive an action of a significant other as unloving at one point in time, such as an uncle arguing with your father, and from another perspective as loving, when at a later point in time you find out that your uncle was trying to prevent a tragic turn of events from taking place.

.You may come to understand a loved one's past hurtful acts as fearful responses to a perceived threat, gaining empathy and compassion for him or her. In some instances, it is not that some aspect of the actual Universe changes, but rather your understanding of it has changed, altering your perceived Universe. In those moments, you may time-travel through internal experience without ever leaving the present to change a perception of the past, present, or future. These trips through time are powerful tools against the illusions of distorted perception.

AMNESIA, HYPERMNESIA, PARAMNESIA, AND CRYTOMNESIA

Amnesia is a hypnotic phenomenon that removes some aspect of the Universe or your psyche from higher levels of conscious awareness. Following such a removal, you are unable to place it back in conscious awareness without a further suggestion or a reorganization of your perceived Universe.

Hypermnesia is the opposite of amnesia, the capability to recall in detail past experience, a heightened memory recall. You are always remembering and forgetting some aspects of your perceived Universe. As I wrote in one of my journal articles:

> In hypermnesia the phenomenal [perceived] field is shifted to a moment in time when a past experience occurred, while all other current aspects of the field of awareness (including physiological, environmental, and psychological aspects) drop into ground.[53]

All of your experiences are mentally recorded or stored, and they are accessible during hypnosis, when they can be brought into your personal world to maximize potential. A forgotten memory is not randomly forgotten, but is buried as a result of your need in the present.

Just as what is forgotten is due to your current need for adequacy, you can later remember the same event when needs change. For example, a man might find it painful to remember the rejection of a loved one; later, however, when the man is stronger, he may be able to process this rejection and grow beyond the limits of his past.

It is also the case that memories may remain in a particular organization of your personal world at higher levels of awareness, while other aspects of life at a vague or low level of awareness cause concern. Changing perception will then become very difficult. If there is something worrisome or anxiety-provoking bothering you, you may concern yourself instead with daily routines and responsibilities, making them the focus of your attention and anxiety instead.

Paramnesia is not being able to tell dreams or fantasies from events that really happened. This kind of experience can occur during hypnosis, under certain conditions such as crytomnesia. Crytomnesia is when something is remembered from the past but believed to be a new and original idea even though it is not. Crytomnesia demonstrates that your mind records and stores every experience that you have, although you may not be able to recall where or when the experiences occurred unless you create context by bringing other aspects of your perceived Universe existent at that time into higher levels of your present awareness. Dreams are so vivid that if a dream you can't remember comes back to you during hypnosis, you could possibly think that the experience actually occurred.

POSITIVE HALLUCINATIONS

Positive hallucinations are things you see that are not present and are thus an illusion. (A delusion differs from an illusion; it is a false belief that a person holds and is unwilling to change, even when opposing evidence is provided.) Hallucinations are not really present in your physical world but are imagined in your subjective and internally perceived Universe. These phenomena have been demonstrated in sensory deprivation experiments,[54] where people hallucinate after having been deprived of visual or auditory stimulation for long periods.

Questions often arise about this phenomenon. How do you determine in everyday life that something is a positive hallucination rather than something actually existent in the physical Universe? How do you know that someone is hallucinating rather than accurately perceiving some other aspects of the Universe? Why do persons reject the experiences of others simply because they have not had similar events in their lives? Does it need to be a *folie à deux* (a rare psychiatric syndrome where symptoms of a delusional belief are transferred from one individual to another) to be considered an accurate perception of reality?

This definition reminds me of how George Orwell, an English novelist and journalist, in his book *Nineteen Eighty Four*, depicts memory reconstruction by institutions for a social consensus, wherein reality-based reconstructed contradictory memories and experiences are interpreted as delusions and hallucinations.[55] Orwell's government of the future establishes an outside authority for defining what constitutes accurate perceiving and what constitutes a problematic view of the external world.

A great ancient example of this attempting to reconstruct memories is the case of St. Joan of Arc. This patron saint of France and saint of the Roman Catholic church was faced with defending the accuracy of her perceptions when dealing with sixty-two learned university and church men who after four trials in 1431 were unable to get this uneducated eighteen-year-old peasant girl, who could not read, to say something that was spiritually damaging about herself. At one point, pro-English Bishop of Beauvais Pierre Cauchon asked her if she heard the voices of the saints, particularly Saint Margaret and Saint Catherine. Joan of Arc responded that she had heard their voices. He then asked her if she was in a state of grace. At this point one of the church clergy, Jean Lefevre, stepped forward protesting that such a question was unfair and too subtle to ask her. It was an intellectual trap, for had she admitted to being in a state of grace, she would have been convicted of heresy. Her brilliant answer left no room for heresy as she stated: "If I am not, may God put me there; and if I am, may God so keep me." For if Joan of Arc truly heard the voices of the saints and was communicating with the divine, Bishop Cauchon, a representative of the church was committing a much graver sin, attempting to make Joan of Arc disbelieve and doubt her own spiritual experiences.

For the French people, Joan sacrificed herself to unite all of France, and for self-righteous Bishop Cauchon, she was a heretic and witch to be burned at the stake, as a mirror only to his own darkness. Like my great-grandfather Chief Madockawando in 1690, St. Joan of Arc in 1431 could not read. Both were read documents by the English and were told what they were signing, while secretly the documents they actually signed were switched and quite different from what they had been told they were signing. In this way, political and religious leaders distorted the truth, hiding their true thoughts and actions with lies and deceit, as they caused harm to two very spiritual human beings with brute physical force and mental games aimed at securing power "money" for themselves.

A variation on the same theme is in Dr. Leo Buscaglia's Animal School, where animals' gifts are damaged by requirements to perform acts unnatural to them. Similarly, in today's world of psychiatry, sometimes medication is prescribed to clients for seeing things a prescriber doesn't perceive. This "solution" does not take into account the possibility that one person could be the only individual who sees something extraordinary that exists in the Universe or in another individual's perceived Universe. Because there are no preset criteria to evaluate such experiences, they are often labeled psychotic, delusional, or magical thinking, despite the possibility that they could potentially be genuinely accurate perceptual experiences, the result of an expanding perceptual awareness of the Universe.

When comparing literature from different fields of study, the controversy over what is accurately perceived can be quite interesting. For instance, consider comparing and contrasting definitions of *magical thinking* and *psychokinesis* (affecting the world around you with your mind). A manual developed by the American Psychiatric

Association (APA) to help professionals determine a person's diagnosis of mental illness defines magical thinking as "The erroneous belief that one's thoughts, words, or actions will cause or prevent a specific outcome in some way that defies commonly understood laws of cause and effect."[56] Notice how this definition of magical thinking intersects with the definition of psychokinesis written by Richard Broughton, a research psychologist: "[Psychokinesis] is the apparent ability of the human being to affect objects, events, or even people around him or her without using the usual intervention by the muscular system."[57] I once knew a woman whose boyfriend visualized winning the lottery every day. He later won the lottery and is receiving $50,000 a year for twenty years. Would this be considered magical thinking? As author Michael Biagent stated:

> For truth, as we have seen, is something to be experienced directly, rather than sought intellectually. . . . It goes without saying to know is always greater than to believe.[58]

Stanley Krippner, an internationally known humanistic psychologist, who has written about shamanism, demonstrated how mental health professionals have equated experiences of shamans with mental illness.[59] Allen Bergin, a clinical psychologist, known for his work on psychotherapy outcome and integrating psychotherapy and religion, offered an interesting definition: "Pathology is that which disturbs the person or those in the environment. The clinician then forms an alliance with the person or society to eliminate the disturbing behavior."[60] Throughout history many scientists with what seemed like radical ideas at the time have "disturbed the environment," such as by discovering the Earth revolves around the Sun and that bacteria exist that you cannot see with your eyes. The few standing against the many might be the only ones who expose lies and reveal truths.

Hallucinations occur for individuals, spontaneously and effortlessly, unfolding as naturally as scenes on a Sunday drive through the countryside. Many people have come to fear that describing their hallucinations, even those in the form of spiritual experiences, will cause others to "think I'm crazy." Such people worry about how others will judge them, while feeling that their experiences are authentic and real and not illusions or fantasies. It is important to realize that delusions are quite different from genuine spiritual experiences; each has unique characteristic features.

Dr. Arthur Combs pointed out that a genuine delusion during a psychotic episode is a function of an individual's distorted self-concept.[61] In such cases, the psychosis is a way for the individual to maximize the potential of the perceived self and, according to Drs. Snygg and Combs, ". . . to deal with the threats" perceived.[62] An example of a psychosis fulfilling a person's needs is reflected in an experience of a client of mine who had been raped and was afraid to speak to a man she found attractive because her primal fear of being attacked was associated with her erotic feelings. She hallucinated conversations with the attractive man because they were "safe," allowing her to believe she had a viable relationship without actually risking physical contact with him. Such complex responses are very individual and are difficult to generalize about.

Similarly, human spiritual experiences that are not delusions are hard to define and even harder to falsify. They differ from psychoses in that they all reveal universal themes of human experiences. More about this subject will be explored in Chapters 9 and 10.

An example of how a positive hallucination might operate in one's perceived Universe during hypnotic experiences is illustrated by a case of Dr. Peter Sheehan's. Using his Experiential Analysis Technique (EAT), Sheehan gave his client a hypnotic suggestion during hypnosis to have a positive hallucination of a friend.[63] During this positive hallucination, the woman had a conversation with her hallucinated friend that involved her being unable to find her contact lenses. Later, Dr. Sheehan removed the suggestion of seeing a friend in the room and believed that he had removed the entire experience as well. Still later, after the hypnosis was over, this woman believed that the contact lenses involved remained on the floor in the room where she had been hypnotized. While Dr. Sheehan removed her hallucinated friend with a hypnotic suggestion, he did not remove the perception of contact lenses, which remained at higher levels of awareness for the woman, even after he brought her out of hypnosis. She was thus unable to reorganize her perceived Universe to what it had been prior to her hypnotic experience. Once Dr. Sheehan became aware of this continued differentiation, he was able to repeat the hypnosis and remove the contact lenses; then the woman returned to the prior organization of her perceived Universe. Although this type of experience is rather rare in hypnosis, it does occur in your everyday life at low levels of awareness and illustrates how your perceptual processes can influence daily life.

NEGATIVE HALLUCINATIONS

Conversely, negative hallucinations involve not seeing things that are aspects of your present Universe, responding as if they do not exist. For example, a person might bump into a wall because it was not seen, ignore what another person has said because the person is not perceived as being there, or dismiss subjective or internal experience such as a bodily sensation that is not sensed. These are often common phenomena in everyday life positioned at low levels of awareness.

For example, a client of mine was unable to find his wallet even though it was in his hand or unable to see a coffee cup right on the table in front of him. Just as he was doing, you do not differentiate some aspects of your perceived Universes as you seek to maintain and maximize your perceived self at a given moment in time.

In the case of the woman client who had been raped, she was unable to see the attractive man when he was actually in the room because she was so frightened; she responded as if he was not there. She placed these aspects of her perceived Universe in low levels of awareness, where they were not brought into figure.

Negative hallucinations can also include a lack of bodily awareness. Sensations of movement, strains to muscles, tendons, or joints can exist outside awareness, as well as our emotions, vibrations, noises, and even others speaking to you. These aspects of the Universe remain located in ground and undifferentiated.

ANALGESIA AND ANESTHESIA

Analgesia, the absence of bodily awareness of pain, and anesthesia, which literally means loss of perceived bodily sensation, may occur in any aspect of your bodily awareness. In such cases, you place a particular aspect of your perceived Universe or self into lower levels of awareness. Many people experience these two phenomena quite often. How many times has a pain or headache vanished when you focused on something else? Or perhaps a cut only began to hurt when you realized you had a skin laceration.

Dr. William Kroger, a pioneer in the use of medical hypnosis, stated that the first reported use of hypnosis to induce anesthesia occurred in 1829 when Dr. Jules Cloquet, a French surgeon, used it to perform a breast amputation.[64] John Elliotson, an English physician, at the University Hospital of London,[65] and his student James Esdaile, a Scottish surgeon,[66] removed pain from their clients' awareness while conducting surgical operations on them before anesthetics such as ether were discovered. The mortality rate for surgery at that time was as high as 25 percent, but Drs. Esdaile and Elliotson reduced it to around 5 percent in their patients! As these physicians nurtured natural internal resources to heal, others raced to develop external resources that in the long term became a part of modern medicine, but to this day introduce risks that hypnosis does not. Had science emphasized hypnosis rather than chemical anesthesia, techniques deploying hypnosis might be common knowledge today and frequently used when preparing patients for surgery. Preparing them to use their minds, rather than simply dealing with their physical being, would perhaps eliminate the extra expense and potential risk of drug-induced anesthesia.

During a time I wore braces on my teeth, my periodontist and orthodontist were amazed that I felt no pain while using my self-hypnosis ability. My cousin, a physician, stated: "Well, that says a lot about your neurological system." Wondering if something was wrong with my bodily ability to feel sensations, I focused on feeling the braces. For the next several days, I had pain and was uncomfortable, which interfered with my concentration and distracted me. It took me several days of imagining the pain being removed to place the discomfort of the braces back into the ground of my experience.

A client reported that after attending a workshop that taught participants self-hypnosis, she was able to go to her dentist and "eliminate pain through self-hypnosis." She reported that her going to the dentist changed from a negative experience with considerable anxiety into a positive and relaxing one. Bodily pain that had previously been so central to her experience went into vague or lower levels of awareness when she reorganized her perceived Universe. Drs. Snygg and Combs further explain:

> In some cases the phenomenal self may even be located outside the body. . . . This effect may also be observed in hypnotized subjects who are subjected to pain-inducing experiences but do not feel pain, apparently because the pain is relegated to the not-self. Since it does not affect the self, it is not experienced.[67]

Without hypnosis, pain naturally brings the affected part of your body into clear figure while placing other aspects into lower levels of awareness. As you change differentiations of your perceived self to include only aspects of bodily awareness that do not include the painful area during hypnosis, the intensity of pain can be reduced.

In some instances aspects of your personal world may be placed at lower levels of awareness, yet continue to influence you in some way. I experienced this phenomenon when I ingested morphine following my serious motorcycle accident as medical personnel straightened out my left leg. My conscious awareness recognized no pain due to the medication. Strangely, I cried out in pain anyway, as the medical staff straightened out my leg, while being consciously puzzled because I did not actually feel any pain. I recognized that some other level of awareness within me had perceived the physical pain and responded. I wondered if that experience was like the phenomenon of automatic talking or writing, in which a person says or writes what is perceived at low levels of awareness. Channeling may be a way of receiving and communicating material that is normally at ground or low level of awareness, and not available at higher levels of awareness. Perhaps the same type of phenomenon occurs for people working on developing psychic intuitive capacities, when thoughts are allowed to flow through the mind unfiltered and they make statements whose source they cannot identify.

POST-HYPNOTIC SUGGESTION

A post-hypnotic suggestion is a suggestion made to you during hypnosis that remains at low levels of awareness in your perceived Universe, even after the hypnotic session ends. This approach can reorganize your perceived Universe. Such a suggestion remains at a low level of awareness while you, coming out of hypnosis, return to a former reorganization of your perceived Universe (as it existed before the post-hypnotic suggestion was given). Suggestions of this sort are later manifested in your behavior; for example, the suggestion to open a window when another person enters a room might result in your taking that action without realizing why. Such phenomena may be similar to phobic reactions—where a person's behavior in the present is a reaction to an imagined memory of an original fearful experience from the past that is typically sustained at low levels of awareness.

Post-hypnotic suggestion readily demonstrates how suggestion is a function of perception, phenomenal field dynamics, and a need to maintain or maximize your potential. It illustrates how, at low levels of awareness, you manifest hypnotic experience in your everyday life—in a way, you are performing post-hypnotic self-suggestions with your thoughts and beliefs. You become what you perceive when particular thoughts stay inside your mind and integrate with your preexisting consciousness.

Post-hypnotic suggestions can be conveyed to you through verbal or nonverbal means, such as words, images, and emotions. Through suggestion, the gestalt of your perceptual awareness is altered, so that you may shiver on a warm day, or not smell ammonia when it is placed under your nose, or eat a raw onion without tearing up.

Post-hypnotic suggestions can result from experience at low levels of awareness in everyday life. You often remain unaware that your perception has taken on meanings at low levels of awareness and that you respond automatically in the present based on past experience. Hypnosis researcher Stanley Fisher, in 1954, pointed out how your perceived meaning of an event or behavior can cause you to act in different ways. He conducted an experiment to demonstrate that subjects carried out post-hypnotic suggestions only when someone was evaluating them.[68] He used the post-hypnotic suggestion that his subjects would scratch their ears when they heard the word psychology. He used several different ways of suggesting this phenomenon to alter their responsiveness, suggesting at one point that the experiment was completed and at another point that he was removing suggestions given during hypnosis. As Kenneth Bowers, PhD and hypnosis researcher, summarized:

> In other words, the subject's ear scratching behavior was turned on and off by the subject's perception of whether the experiment was on or off. This result contrasts rather dramatically with the credulous view that hypnotic subjects invariably respond in a literal and compulsive fashion to post-hypnotic suggestions.[69]

Drs. Fisher's and Bowers's findings reveal that it is mainly your individual personal meanings and perceptions that determine your responses to suggestions and other hypnotic techniques. Within hypnotic experience you find an answer to the riddle of the undiscovered dynamics of perceptual awareness in everyday life!

You create your reality in relation to how you perceive the world. This fact is supported by the placebo effect. One case illustrating the placebo effect was of a patient whose illness went into remission when he believed his cancer medication was proven effective and then returned after he heard news reports of a study that showed his medication's lack of effectiveness. Fortunately, the treatment was again found effective and hearing that put the patient's illness into remission once again.[70] Such cases point to the possibility that much of the information and news you hear falsely creates or removes possibilities in your life, without you even knowing that such suggestions had any impact.

A myth voiced by one individual during a survey was: "It's well known that a hypnotic suggestion only lasts for a short time before it loses its effect." I would not be so quick to make such a statement. For example, you may have a dream tonight about a stranger, and then seven years from now meet that person exactly as he or she appeared in your dream. A shamanic counselor I know told me her sister-in-law, at the age of twelve, dreamt that she was marrying a young man whose identical self stood next to him at the church altar. She ended up marrying the counselor's brother, whose twin was the best man on the altar! About a dozen years after the dream. Such experiences suggest that time is irrelevant in certain instances, as suggestions and expanded consciousness demonstrate. Will you remember that dream and make the connection between it and this current encounter? You will probably not remember your dreams for that long. Back in 1964, Hans Eysenck, a British psychologist born in Germany stated: "Responsible investigators have claimed that post-hypnotic suggestions have been carried out as many as five years after they were originally given."[71]

CATALEPSY

Catalepsy is a hypnotic phenomenon in which you are unable to move a particular part of your body, such as an eyelid or an arm. Bodily awareness of that aspect of your perceived self has simply been placed into lower levels of awareness and thus restricted your self-definition. During catalepsy, you typically will not bring those body parts of your perceived self into higher levels of awareness until your personal world reverts to the experience that existed prior to the catalepsy. If you cannot imagine your arms as moving, then your arms will remain immobile during hypnosis. Hypnosis may further enhance immobility by removing any images or thoughts that are subjectively counteractive to the desired effect.

Beyond this phenomenon, a perceptual model of hypnosis implies that the fatigue or pain of the physical body has gone into ground through reorganization of the phenomenal field so that you do not perceive the fatigue, pain, or that part of your physical body. This is the result of a restricted self-definition. This model also takes into account the possibility that the absence of pain or fatigue can be seen as fulfilling the need for adequacy.[72]

SUBCONSCIOUS MANIFESTATIONS

Subconscious manifestations are behaviors that result from aspects of your personal world that you have relegated to a low level of awareness. One example, ideomotor action, is a phenomenon where a subject makes motions "unconsciously." You might have had ideomotor responses when, for instance, you imagined pain and your body reacted reflexively to the idea alone, without actually undergoing a traumatic blow or condition. You might also produce tears in reaction to powerful emotions without realizing it.

One way to explain ideomotor actions could be by seeing them as a hypnotic phenomenon manifested as behavior derived from low levels of internal awareness. In a hypnotic session, the hypnotist suggests a specific body movement to convey agreement or disagreement with his or her guiding words; for example, an involuntary movement of your little finger to express disagreement. You may have spontaneous movements and perceptions that convince you that something is going on during hypnosis that is not what you normally experience in your perceived Universe. For example, you might not be aware of the hypnotic experience, as if you were sleeping, but then wake up at the count of three as if some other part of your awareness were listening the entire time.

Another example of subconscious manifestation is responding to an instruction to completely focus on studying for school and forget everything around you. You later find while multitasking and studying that you suddenly cannot remember the tasks that you have been carrying out other than studying. This phenomenon of subconscious manifestation has implications for such concepts as psychosomatic problems—perhaps you have seen it in your own life when you or someone you know has developed physical suffering as a means of expressing emotional or psychological pain.

SOMNAMBULISM

Somnambulism (also called sleepwalking) is the deepest state of hypnosis reported and used by one of Mesmer's followers, Armand-Marie-Jacques de Chastenet, Marquis of Puységur, a French aristocrat who was able to hypnotize some subjects so deeply that they were able to diagnose illnesses in others. A person in this state might walk around with eyes open and talk with the hypnotist. The person may have a fixated attention and slowed or slurred speech, the only indicators that the person is not actually awake and conscious.

As a hypnotic phenomenon, somnambulism manifests an alternate organization of a one's personal world through altered levels of awareness, often involving amnesia or two separate perceived Universes that appear to be mutually exclusive.

In other words, the person does not seem to remember when conscious groups of experiences that happen when in the somnambulistic level of awareness and remembers only the somnambulistic experiences when in that particular organization of awareness. Such hypnotic phenomena could be important in understanding multiple personalities and the complex functioning of personality in everyday life.

During altered awareness while undergoing hypnosis, you might remember every past experience of hypnosis or everything else about past events in everyday life. Then, on terminating the hypnosis, you may not recall that particular hypnotic occurrence, no matter how much conscious effort you exert. People are normally aware of all their experiences in hypnosis, unless they are in a very deep level of hypnosis. Such inaccessible differentiations demonstrate that a reorganization of your perceived Universe has taken place.

As you can see, examining hypnotic phenomena can help you to gain greater control over your hidden and creative potential. Becoming familiar with the specific types of hypnotic phenomena helps you understand hypnosis more and removes its tendency to seem mysterious. These phenomena help you understand that your Universe is shaped by what you choose to accurately perceive and creatively imagine. Ultimately, you choose to either maintain or expand your Universe and your personal meanings.

PERCEPTUAL POINTS

Hypnotic phenomena such as amnesia, hypermnesia, paramnesia, and crytomnesia can be explained perceptually.

- The perceptual dynamics of positive and negative hallucinations are presented.
- The perceptual process of analgesia and anesthesia are outlined.
- The time aspects of post hypnotic suggestions are pointed out.
- From a perceptual view we explain catalepsy, subconscious manifestations, and somnambulism. For example, you may speed up and slow down the subjective experience of time through altering perceptual awareness.
- As you move more aspects of a past experience into higher levels of awareness, you begin to relive the past as it occurred at a particular moment in time.
- You often remain unaware that your perceptions have taken on meanings at low levels of awareness and that you respond automatically in the present based on past experience.

PERCEPTUAL EXERCISE

Take a particular behavior or past experience and come up with as many different ways of viewing that behavior or experience as you can over the course of a few days. If you have someone you trust in your life, ask that person to add to the list. Or take an event, such as a dinner party, a spectator event or concert, or even a conversation between several people. Try to see it from each person's point of view. Start with your own point of view. Then try to look at it from your friend's point of view, perhaps a family member's, and maybe even your cat's or dog's. In this way, you are expanding your perceptual possibilities by reorganizing your perceived Universe.

CHAPTER SEVEN

CHANGING YOUR PERCEPTIONS—RELATING

There's always a different way of viewing anything, no matter how absolute it is.[73]

—*Dr. Milton Erickson*

We perceive more accurately as we expand our awareness of ourselves and our relationship to the limitless aspects of the Universe. Our relationships with others are rich and rewarding ways to perceive new aspects of ourselves. Often others can see what we cannot. Just like individual experiences, others can help us expand or restrict our perceptual awareness. One of the goals of all forms of hypnotic experiences and spirituality is to perceive the world and our life as accurately as possible in relationship to others. The less aware we are, the more self-absorbed we are in daily life, as the connection between ourselves and the Universe remains undifferentiated.

PERCEPTION IS RELATIONAL

Other people are more than merely mirrors of the self, and you must avoid the philosophical trap of solipsism, that ancient philosophical notion that you are alone in the Universe and everything else is a figment of your imagination—that everything you see is just in your mind. Such a state of being narrows your personal world to just the perceived self and internal experiences, and is oblivious to any outside influence.

According to this view, for example, you cannot love or hate something about another person unless it reflects something that you love or hate about yourself. This view ignores the connections to positive external influences in the Universe and effectively shuts down your perceptual awareness. Such a concept of existence, where all is just a matter of self-reflection, leads only to distorted perceptions and illusions. It is reminiscent of the story of Narcissus, the youth of Greek mythology, who fell in love with and wished to rejoin his own image reflected in the water of a lake. When others love you, you hope they love you for who you are with all your imperfections rather than for simply a self-created image of you that is an extension of them.

It is important how you relate to others. When you treat living beings as "objects," others remain undifferentiated. In this way, you dehumanize yourself in the process. For example, completely ignoring another person(s) is as violent an act as physically abusing them. However, such nonphysical violence against others cannot easily be measured and tends to go unreported and under-examined. Harming another is the same as harming yourself.

CHANGING PERCEPTIONS THROUGH RELATIONSHIPS

A shared goal of both spiritual experiences and hypnosis is changing perception, especially those aspects of your perceived Universe that are inaccurate. Two ways of rationalizing distorted perception are by attracting others who see the world the same way and by seeking similar experiences. Thus you might pick the same type of friends, mates, and work, searching for people who support your distorted perception. Changing perceptions and seeking new experiences may sometimes be scary because you cannot always fall back on your past experiences to understand what is happening in the moment. Sometimes changing perception involves experiencing a threat and mourning the loss of old aspects of your perceived Universe as they fade away while new differentiations come into figure.

Let's look at a story that illustrates distorted perceiving. A fatigued person driving along a country road sees something moving in the middle of the road and fears that it is an injured animal. Ninety-nine times out of a hundred it is a garbage bag, tree branch, or other debris. From the time when the person first spots this object to the moment he or she actually identifies it, he or she remains convinced that it is an injured animal. Chances are you can remember a time when something like this happened to you.

You feel generally safe with familiar experiences. You try to put new events into perspective through relating them to past ones. When you cannot compare present perceptions to past experience, you must learn new ways of accurately perceiving others, your Universe, and yourself. This is one reason why you might fear entering hypnosis for the first time. Hypnotic experience involves embracing the unknown and uncertainty. Your self-concept or your more permanent self-definitions determine what you differentiate and how you see yourself. Drs. Snygg and Combs explained that your phenomenal self expresses your relationship to the Universe.[74]

Your perceived self consists of many self-definitions. These various aspects of your perceived self will shift in and out of your perceptual awareness at any particular moment. The more adequate you feel, the more likely you will be able to accept changing views of self and new experiences.

Personal meanings are of utmost importance in this context. A client of mine, who was acquainted with a very attractive woman, refused to ask her out because he saw her with a male friend he believed to be successful and single. In reality this other male was a married lawyer and just her platonic friend, and the woman was available for dating. Uncovering the truth changed his view of the Universe. Most clients of hypnosis report that hypnosis definitely changes the way they see themselves, others in their lives, and the world around them. Learning to perceive in different ways is sometimes difficult but also necessary to expand your perceived Universe.

How you feel is a function of your perception, and hypnosis can help you to make healthy changes in both areas. What you externally express and what you internally experience can be two entirely different things. How you perceive self, others, and the Universe are predictors of how you will behave in any given situation. One of the goals of perceptual hypnosis is to enhance the differentiation process by changing perception or personal meanings. As a result you can (and many clients do) conclude treatment in a shorter period of time using hypnosis than with other therapies, because immediate or gradual differentiations may be utilized to improve a situation quite readily.

Our actions are expressions of personal meaning that lie much deeper. For example, a twenty-six-year-old Caucasian female came to me for help with her compulsive eating. She was healthy, athletic, in good physical condition, and just slightly overweight. At our third session, she said, "It's amazing; I've seen a psychiatrist for six months, and then a psychologist for six months. Neither one of them helped me. With two sessions of hypnosis with you, I now know what my real problem has been. I want to have a baby." She was able to perceive the real conflict and work out her own solution to the problem through hypnosis by getting in touch with her own internal experience.

Another former client was a teenage male who moved from a country town to a city school and could not manage his anxiety about the changes he experienced in this move. As a result, his athletic performance also suffered. By removing his perceived anxiety that distorted his perception in regards to other people, his sense of self was able to actualize his potential more quickly and easily. After a session with perceptual hypnosis, he hit three home runs and brought his superior performance back through achievement of higher levels of awareness.

REMOVING DISTORTED PERCEPTION IN RELATIONSHIPS

In society, relationships have increasingly become dependent on the spoken and written word, even when some experiences defy such modes of expression. The written and spoken word can be more easily manipulated than other forms of communication. This dependency gives rise to distorted perception, as you become accustomed to and accept discrepancies between what you experience and what others determine your experiences mean. Even with your friends, you often respond to their reports of experiences as if an obviously distorted perception is not part of the account. A client of mine quit her job due to ethical concerns over quality assurance. While visiting a friend of hers, she read a text from a mutual friend who thought my client had left her job because of drug or alcohol abuse. This comment could be believed by others and begin rumors. This unfounded comment also hurt her feelings and negatively affected her sense of self. Such distortions can lead to simple misunderstandings or have more serious consequences.

The distortion of communication easily happens in many situations. People communicate perceived threat through their actions or ignore perceived threat through lack of action. Residential home staff reported feeling unsafe at a facility for adolescent boys because on one occasion several residents ran around the facility at night with bricks and sticks. On another occasion, the same residents stole a van and went for a joy ride. Staffing was not increased, however, until two adolescent boys assaulted a female staff member in an office. Only when this woman was raped, beaten, and later died did the public become involved in this situation. There were warning signs that the administration did not heed that could have prevented this atrocity. The adolescents themselves had already begun perceiving the situation at the facility as unsafe and, therefore, had started acting out.

This battle of seeing through distorted perceptions to perceive more accurately has been a major theme throughout history. And any story, great or small, is usually a symbolic version of everyday life struggles for each of us. In the Dead Sea Scrolls there is reference to a conflict between the Priest of Deceit and the Teacher of Righteousness, the latter driven into exile. History is full of murder and betrayal, situations in which rightful kings and queens and other leaders lost their thrones to murderers and deceivers who then controlled the knowledge given to the masses. Seeing accurately means seeing through these deceptions and lies spread by the unworthy to advance themselves unjustly.

These types of events do not occur only in fiction; they have occurred throughout human history. In 2012, in the country of Cote d'Ivoire' in the town of Divo, the village of Gbalouville remains without a chief, as the last chief's son stays in hiding because of numerous attempts on his life. He has even had to protect himself spiritually from attacks in the night of what they call *Marabouts*, spirits that try to harm people in their sleep. He has experienced jealousy from would-be competitors and there have been attempts at poisoning his food. When he was a child, his father did not want him to leave his village for fear of harm coming to him from sorcerers. His maternal grandparents, who were ruling a nearby village, did not want his nuclear family in power. Tchétché Jules was the original chief of this village and his oldest son, Tchétché Gbalou Philipe, followed as chief but died as a result of the jealousy of his uncles and the complicity of his brother. Chief Tchétché Gbalou Philipe was murdered. This is a true story of murder and betrayal.

On the opposite side of the coin, a rare mystic may see reality for what it truly is without any degree of distorted perception, even if only momentarily. As Dr. Abraham Maslow, an American psychologist who created the hierarchy of needs stated: "A single glimpse of heaven is enough to confirm its existence even if it is never experienced again."[75] Hypnosis helps to filter out distorted personal meanings and allows you to come to grips with discrepancies in your life so that you may respond to your world more effectively.

RESTRICTING PERCEPTIONS THROUGH RELATIONSHIPS

When a person sees self in an inadequate way, he often treats others in a negative manner. For example, someone who continually talks about others behind their backs may soon begin to worry that others are talking about him or her. Similarly, people who are constantly attempting to take advantage of those around them for material gain will worry about others doing the same to them. Worry is the negative use of imagination, but it can lead to positive change. Feelings of inadequacy that fuel the practice of gossip and talking about others behind their backs usually stem from a perceived threat to one's self. As individuals begin to see themselves in a more positive light, they no longer engage in conversations of this sort. Thus they no longer feel concerned about what others are saying about them.

You develop a viewpoint or series of perceptions of the world. You use these perceptions to live and understand the world and personal experiences. A new experience that does not fit into this established viewpoint forces you to expand your perceptual field to incorporate that experience into your viewpoint. This expansion creates new perceptions that, in turn, create new behavior. Changes, whether involuntary, such as losing your job, or voluntary, such as bringing new people and experiences into your perceived Universe, and/or altering your perception of yourself through acquiring new skills and abilities, can expand your perceived Universe. The world around you is changing and evolving daily. The more accurately you can perceive your Universe, the more adequate the adjustment you can make to your world. For example, you may see the good in someone, despite the person's negative behavior.

Some people restrict their perceived Universe in order to reject new experiences and maintain an old point of view or rigid perceptions and behavior. This rejection is another way we restrict our relationships with other people. For example, if a person were to perceive the Universe only in one color—say, blue—everything would be perceived as blue, such as people, places, and things. If one day this individual perceived a red rose, he or she would either have to change the perceived Universe to now include red or have to place this red object into a low or "unconscious" level of awareness, pretending this experience never happened, and all things are still blue. Many ideologies and groups, and even some areas of psychology, foster this manner of perceiving the Universe! For example, some fundamentalist Christians perceive the Catholic practice of praying to Mary, the mother of Jesus, as worshipping idols. Others consider the practice of Wicca as worshipping the devil. To some of these fundamentalists, those who say they have seen the ghosts of their relatives or experienced telepathy are perceived as having had hallucinations, because some individuals cannot accept that a ghost might exist or a mind can do such things. While beliefs can restrict perceived awareness of the Universe, such points of view cannot alter the truth, whether seen or unseen. A destructive act perpetrated because of a different point of view may be the very act of evil a person is attempting to avoid to remain in line with individual or group beliefs.

UNIQUENESS IN PERCEPTION

As an individual, you bring psychological uniqueness to perception in your relationships. That uniqueness limits your understanding of another's perception. You might know of persons who report hearing the voice of a dead grandmother, a guardian angel, a spiritual guide, or an alien. Such an external source could tell you something about an immediate danger that can then be avoided or provide you with information that helps you solve an existing problem. The actual source of the information does not matter, as long as the perception or personal meaning presented is acceptable to the recipient, such as angels for Christians or aliens for astronomers. The key is these experiences are in synch with the peoples' lives and help them adapt more adequately, unlike the situation of psychotics whose voices and hallucinations only cause to harm and endanger them or others.

As an individual you can experience color, as you can any other aspect of the Universe, uniquely—having your own response to its appearance and assigning it your own meaning. However, even color may communicate relationship issues in human interaction. For example, a therapist who was a client of mine dreamed about a suspect acquaintance of his who had an identical twin in his dream. That twin of the acquaintance gave a sense of foreboding to the dreaming therapist and appeared as all blue. Bright blue generally is a spiritual color, often related to communication in dreams, and electric blue was the dreamer's favorite color. Still, this bright blue appearance did not feel positive in nature to him. Soon after, a new client came to this therapist's office for a few sessions. She described seeing things all blue and attributed it to a spiritual omen from her religious beliefs. The therapist soon realized that there was a connection between his new female client and this blue identical twin in his dream.

As the therapist completed hypnotherapy with this client, she proposed a working relationship, just as the acquaintance with the blue twin had done earlier. Neither individual had any real contribution to offer for business. He realized that after he had sacrificed and worked hard to obtain a quality education in order to make the world a better place, he had found an individual just like the twin he dreamed about, who sought to use his talents for their mutual gain, and that was their connection. Both of them (the dream twin and the client) had similar difficulties with interpersonal relationships and perceiving the genuine needs of others without self-gain. The point is that any phenomenon, in this case a color, can have unique individual meanings in relationships that far outweigh any general meaning ascribed to it. This story demonstrates how applying cookie-cutter approaches, techniques, and general meanings to everyone fails to take into account how each person differentiates a unique personal meaning to persons, places, and things that might contradict common generalized meanings.

Another psychological limitation to accurately perceiving in relationships is the act of projecting your own past experiences onto future experiences of others and those of yourself. For example, while attending college I was tired and exhausted one day because I had stayed awake all night to study for a final exam. As I went through the day, people from all areas of my life responded to my physical appearance of being tired by alluding to their own experiences: "Did you have trouble sleeping last night?" "You must have had a good time—who was she?" "Were you out partying and drinking last night?" Such questions reflected each person's life experience. Only other students who were taking the test recognized that I might have been studying for a test. These individuals perceived my tiredness from their own point of view or frame of reference.

Food has many meanings that remain to be explored. For example, for some it is a way to nurture the self. For others, consuming food brings nonsexual bodily pleasures or lets them demonstrate the ability to outconsume others. Or eating can be a way to return to childhood experiences, where others provided for one's basic needs. For some, food represents economic power or personal control. Through whatever lens one sees food, it is its personal meaning that affects behavior and can affect others.

The simple act of changing your perspective and seeing people or events in different contexts is a powerful creative perceptual force. If we can allow ourselves to see new interactions and connections in the different situations we encounter, we can expand our understanding of the Universe. For example, an insight might make you realize that an overgeneralization such as "all men are insensitive" is not true. Or an event could occur that makes you realize that cause and effect are not the only way that the Universe operates. For example, I encountered an old client of mine at the post office. She asked when I was getting my new puppy. I told her that I had put a nonrefundable deposit down on a pure-black German shepherd puppy and asked the breeder to handpick the right puppy for me. The woman responded, "Oh, you won't get your dog for two years." The client did not know who I had chosen for a breeder. Despite every attempt to get my puppy earlier, the puppy was chosen exactly two years later, to the weekend. So many meaningful coincidences occur that point to an order in the Universe quite different than the one we have been taught to use in everyday life.

Consider, for instance, that a teacher might perceive a creative child as a problem in the classroom environment. Yet, when the child is placed in a social situation, both adults and other children perceive this child as a positive influence whose imagination contributes to an effective leadership style. So it is not solely the child's behavior that creates these differing perceptions. Perceptions of the child cannot be separated from the environment and vary for each individual doing the perceiving. All these points demonstrate how perception is hypnotic in that it creates or distorts how you see the world you live in and how you relate to others. You respond to the Universe based on your perceptual and personal meanings, which cause changes in relating. To change perceptions through hypnotic experience is to change your behavior, yourself, and your relationships with others.

CHANGE IS IN RELATIONSHIP TO LOVE AND FEAR

All experience is grounded in the relationship of self to the Universe. Love is one of the many aspects of relationships that is difficult to measure. To love another, you must be able to enter into a shared space with that person and experience some aspects of the perceived Universe of that person. You must be able to reach out and connect to something other than yourself. Leo Buscaglia, known as Dr. Love, an author and professor at University of Southern California, used the analogy that love is similar to a mirror. In other words, we get what we put into life.[76] However, in the movie *Practical Magic*, actress Sandra Bullock stated it nicely when she said: "I want to be seen." In other words, to love someone is to see them for who they really are, rather than who you wish they were or want them to be.

Loving yourself in another is not the same as authentically loving another human being. If you love only what you see as yourself in another person, then you really are not seeing or loving another person but rather seeing and loving a reflection of what you want to see. You, like anyone, distort your perceptions to some degree. You must acknowledge another's perceptual awareness of you. At first, this task appears to be simple, but on closer examination you find that perceiving the truth of reality accurately is quite difficult. You may choose not to see universal truth, thinking you can bypass it by creating your own reality or personal truth. You tend to see what is best for you, regardless of whether this is based on illusion or an accurate perception of reality. Just as fear narrows your experience of the world, perceived love opens up your worldview. Whether you experience aloneness or love, you must expand the self to understand the aloneness of others or to share love with others. By expanding the self, perceptual hypnosis helps you see your relatedness to people, events, and things; seeing that relationship is necessary in order to experience the world beyond self-indulgence and to move between different viewpoints. For instance, you might as a result of hypnosis realize that when someone genuinely smiles at you, that person is looking at you and acknowledging you as you are. Through realizations like this one, hypnotic experience affirms that perceptual awareness involves relating to all aspects of the Universe, even if some aspects exist only at low levels of awareness.

At the opposite end of the spectrum from love is the perception of separateness from others. Is that perceived separation from one another and closing off others from your worldview an illusion that disconnects you from your spiritual roots and true essence of oneness? And is that separation something that damaged persons teach others? To "love your neighbors as yourself" requires union rather than separation and how you impact others impacts you.

Through hypnosis you take a closer look at how you perceive others and yourself. How you perceive yourself affects not only how you perceive others, but how others perceive you. In a perceptual frame of reference, if you behave as though you are talented, attractive, and successful, then others will be more likely to perceive you that way.

Not only can others enhance or restrict your self-definition by how they perceive you, but you can enhance or restrict another's self-definition when you identify with him or her and respond to that person as attractive. You can place him or her in the background of your perceived Universe based on either attractiveness or unattractiveness. You might place a person in the background if you find that person either unattractive or so attractive that he or she poses a threat to your need to maximize your own potential.

ANGER AS INTERNAL HYPNOTIC PHENOMENA

Perceptual hypnosis can also effectively treat conflict in interpersonal relationships, especially the problem of anger in your life, because a change in internal experience can affect the way you see and relate to others and the surrounding world. Anger is mostly expressed in relationship to others. During moments of anger, your perceived Universe shrinks. Often, even the physical body is perceived in lower levels of awareness. When you are an angry person, you are restricting perceptual awareness through hypnotic phenomena that include:

- Age regression (reliving a past experience in your current relationship— possibly even reverting to childhood behaviors)
- Negative hallucination (not even seeing the other person present in the argument)
- Pseudo-orientation in time (for example, imagining catastrophic future events or reliving past hurts)
- Amnesia (forgetting positive experiences with that person)
- Time distortion (acting as if there is no more time to resolve this situation)

Both male and female perpetrators of domestic violence report experiencing these hypnotic phenomena during their interpersonal conflicts with partners. As a result they might distort their current situations in negative ways. Often the angry person sees himself as out of control and powerless in relationship to significant others and, therefore, acts in ways that are considered power grabbing and controlling behaviors. Altering perception alters these adverse behaviors.

PERCEPTUAL POINTS

- Perceptual hypnosis may bypass distorted cognitive processes that have limited your awareness of other people by helping you see personal meanings in new ways that are unique and develop new differentiations that enhance your relationships and expand your Universe.
- To perceive clearly in the present, you may need to remove yourself from a cloud of personal history created in your interpersonal relationships that may have distorted perceptual awareness in the past.
- By changing your perceptions, you can reduce or eliminate anger and stop power- and control-driven behaviors in relationships.

PERCEPTUAL EXERCISE

Try saying things in new ways. Words have certainly limited your way of relating and may even shape what you do think about relating in a restrictive manner. Try using new creative approaches to words, like using active language rather than describing experience as an unchanging noun so that you bring new views to your life. For example, consider "I am having a great time this summer," rather than "Summer was a great time." Pay attention to the words you use and statements you make, and notice how your language can help shape your experiences. Try to stay in the present. Our life experiences are not a bunch of frozen moments like photographs but rather constitute an active ever-changing process that is continually being altered.

You can utilize your imagination to free you from a restricted inability to differentiate accurately in new ways and to prevent maintaining past distorted perceptions by expanding your awareness. Try finding examples of different meanings in words or images for you and someone close to you, such as a family member, lover, relative, or friend. For one person, "relaxed" may mean listening to rock music, and for another it may be having no noise in the environment at all. See how your uniqueness affects the way you differentiate aspects of the Universe.

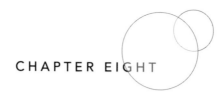

CHAPTER EIGHT

EXTERNAL INFLUENCES: MONEY, MEDIA, AND MIND CONTROL

In these, the status quo, the mores, institutions, morals, status relationships, etc. will come most near to [being so] self-evident that the individual is conformed of himself to them from lack of psychological individuation.[77]

—Dr. James W. Woodard

Every day as you move through your world, you are bombarded with external influences that attempt to subliminally shape your subconscious mind and affect your body, too. Some attempt to get you to spend your money in a specific manner. Others seek to persuade you to behave in certain ways, such as voting for this candidate or acting on a cause. Well-meaning people attempt to create memories for you and manipulate your ways of looking at certain past experiences and current events. They seek to change how you perceive your world.

Perceptual hypnosis helps you stop being influenced adversely by these outside forces. How? It helps you see the world more accurately, thus making you aware of techniques others use to impact you for their own gain. As a result, you can make more informed decisions on what is in your best interest.

By choosing to become conscious of the dynamics of perceptual awareness, you can protect yourself from being unsuspectingly influenced by perceptions fed to you that you then might hold at lower levels of awareness in your mind. You must protect yourself from unknown harm, or you will become a volunteer victim of these external influences. I once met a man I would call an energy vampire who stated he could steal energy because it's a universal right, as he put it. He went on, "People don't protect themselves and so it's their own fault, not mine." His very existence demonstrates there are influences out there we need to protect ourselves against through greater awareness.

A PERCEPTUAL APPROACH TO MONEY THROUGH HYPNOSIS

Since hypnosis can help you with your tendency to be influenced by external forces, and since money is one symbol of those forces, hypnosis can help you relate better to your money. Your relationship to money mirrors your personal meanings in everyday life. Typically, money is an important aspect of your perceived Universe, and its use or misuse is determined by how a given self is perceived in relationship to others and the Universe. Money has many meanings to people. For instance, when money is a component in giving and receiving, its use reflects your perceptions of yourself and the nature of your relationships. Gifts are given for any number of reasons. Some of these reasons may be simple, direct, and altruistic. Money can be given as a gift in an expression of pure generosity. Or it can be given according to a deal, in exchange for something else. There may be more complex motivations behind your monetary interactions; these motives might be in lower levels of consciousness. Some people may use currency to:

- Obtain self-recognition; change your image in your own eyes.
- Receive something back from another indirectly—in other words by manipulation.
- Put another in debt to self as a way to control the other.
- Gain acknowledgment from others.

These motives are more apparent in business relationships. For example, pharmaceutical drug companies often provide free luncheons or other inducements to health professionals to help gain their support in marketing the company's drugs. The exchange of money or gifts of monetary value inevitably affects the ethics of a relationship. There are unspoken dynamics at play in many transactions. The only true gift is that gift which is genuinely given with no strings attached, and no hidden attempts to influence. Are you aware of the nature of your monetary interactions as they occur each day? How about a birthday present to your niece, a tip for a waiter, a payment of alimony or child support, tax estimates, paying off debt, buying a luxury car? What are the inter- and intrapersonal dynamics going on in these scenarios?

Money is often of primary importance in your subjective experiences, especially relationships, yet its implications are rarely considered. Dr. Linn F. Cooper and Dr. Milton Erickson, physicians, described a client, referred to as D, making a statement that is covertly about money:

> D, a neighbor in Yankton, was calling to her little girl, "Don't run. You'll hurt yourself." I felt sorry for the little girl, for I thought "She's [D is] not afraid she'll hurt herself; she's just afraid she'll get her white shoes dirty." And then they will have to be replaced and this costs money.[78]

This is an excellent example of the impact of one person's perceptions hypnotically influencing her child in everyday life. It is also an instance of fear about financial security coloring one of many aspects of one's world. This little girl's future overcautious behaviors may stem from her mother's anxiety about money, which was expressed repeatedly when cautioning her daughter not to hurt herself. The daughter would likely grow to perceive the world as unsafe as a consequence of her mother placing frightening aspects of the Universe into high levels of awareness.

Another example of the hidden influence of money is the expression used in characterizing another's death—"cashing in early." Or you can describe a hectic schedule as "time is money." You have heard these words, words that paint pictures or create visualizations in your mind and affect your behaviors, often unconsciously.

Jerome Bruner, a prominent psychologist teaching at Harvard University, and co-author Cecile Goodman demonstrated, in 1947, that children from poor homes perceived a nickel as the size of a half dollar, and those from affluent homes perceived a half dollar as the size of a nickel.[79] Perceptual hypnosis can help you to become aware of these viewpoints, take a more conscious look at yourself and your behaviors, and change your relationship to money. How persons attain and use money reflects who they truly are as human beings and how they relate to others in their world.

Your perception or image of money can elicit your characteristic manner of perceiving or imagining. A bumper sticker I once saw read, "Jesus Christ—he paid the price." How ironic, since Jesus was angered by the exchange of money in temples. And, for him, worldly possessions meant so little.

Your perceptual awareness of money influences your feelings, thoughts, and behavior, and while such perceptions may occur at low levels of awareness, your actions are partly a response to all the ways you view money's impact on your world. It is also interesting how unsuccessful marriages often begin with love and end in a battle over money.

To understand how you respond to money, you must first ascertain its personal meaning for you. When necessary, you sometimes need to change the irrational and thus distorted perceptions of money you learned from past experiences and come to view it in a more realistic light as simply a medium of exchange. How do you define money? Is it the root of all evil? Do you think you deserve to receive as much money as you require? Some people believe that there are enough financial resources for everyone in the Universe. Others do not want to share their money. Some feel shame in having too much. It is rare to read any authentic disclosures on the personal meaning of money, because the true meaning many place on it remains so hidden. You might consider your finances or discussions of them such a private matter that you never really talk about them and as a result never really analyze how much money influences your decisions.

Large therapeutic service organizations can be heavily influenced by administrative views on money rather than therapeutic considerations alone. Often this detrimentally affects individual clients. A former supervisor of mine related a story about treating an eighteen-year-old Native American Indian female when he was working at a mental health clinic. After extensive psychological testing, he could find no diagnosis for her. The clinical director of the institution told him that he had to give this young woman a diagnosis, despite finding her lacking any mental illness. Later, when this young woman was observed disagreeing with a nurse, she was placed in arm and leg restraints on a bed and medicated, despite the lack of a diagnosis for her. My former supervisor was being pressured to diagnose this individual as mentally ill in order for the institution to receive monetary compensation. A highly ethical psychologist, he reported this episode to the state's mental health board. Subsequently, that clinical director and nurse were dismissed from their jobs. When he later told this story to licensed psychologists, master's level licensed clinicians, clinical trainees, and interns, many responded by saying, "I would have just given her a diagnosis." Such a decision is deplorable—an instance where money compromises ethics and an abuse of power is motivated by money.

Some individuals are exploited by people who alter their personal meanings and perception of money. An exploiter influences a "victim's" perceptions to essentially change that person's views to fit the exploiter's vision for the use of money. Such individuals distract their "victims" from the essential truth or accurate view of a situation by drawing their attention or shifting their focus to unessential aspects. The perpetrator influences their victims' perceptions and their need for adequacy in a hypnotic manner. These perpetrators, whom I call "vampires," are like parasites that do not include the well-being of others as part of their self-definitions. These vampires tend to target individuals who have money for them to steal. Your journey using perceptual hypnosis can help you avoid becoming a victim of a vampire. Even when you are able to examine and acknowledge your vulnerabilities, weaknesses, and mistakes, there are always people in the world who attempt to exploit your foibles for their own gain. So you do need to be more aware and to protect yourself.

Meanwhile, individuals with poor self-images and little or no money often remain unnoticed or are attended to at low levels of awareness during interpersonal communications in human society, due to their being perceived as lacking resources and as being unsuitable in varying ways, as either friends or victims. On the flip side, such individuals don't often believe they deserve success. As a result, many do not perceive money and its benefits as part of their self-definition. The effects of these people having less money and having lower levels of achievement serve to demonstrate how you attract and repel what you perceive or choose not to perceive, both in everyday perceptual awareness and hypnosis. Your perceptual awareness is like a magnet, drawing particular aspects of the Universe toward you and repelling other aspects away from you.

Of course, your perceptions of money and its impact may be misleading or distorted, but it is what you have failed to differentiate in your perceived Universe that creates this distortion. To further complicate the Universe, unclear perceptions tend to disable positive attractions. As Donald Snygg said: ". . . a highly detailed and differentiated field will include definite and precise behavior, while, as anyone who has tried to find a light switch in a strange room in the dark will agree, behavior in a vague and undifferentiated field is vague and confused."[80] You need to bring into differentiation a more detailed understanding of the psychological meaning of money. When you exchange money with someone else, you tend toward either enhancing each other's needs or neutralizing each other's resources. This is done based on one's sense of personal adequacy and the adequacy of the other.

An understanding of the significance of the need for adequacy, and granting it to others, would lead society to distribute resources differently. How persons attain and use money symbolizes who they truly are as human beings and how they relate to others in their world. Helping people develop adequacy requires addressing:

- Poor and crowded housing
- Nutritional deficiencies
- Medical neglect
- Unemployment

And these remedies are only a start for people struggling on the inadequate side of the continuum. In turn, this type of societal change can only happen when large numbers of people in society enter a shared space and identify with others, perceiving them as significant in their Universes. That persons in the United States, or in any advanced nation, are left dying and suffering because they lack money for medicine and healthcare remains at low levels of awareness. The American culture of immediate self-gratification—focused on what you can gain right now—is based on a rigid and inflexible perceived self and Universe.

I recently observed an ATM from which one can gain instant access to money— in a local bar! So as you drink more alcohol and your ability to control your impulses diminishes, you can have instant access to your cash and spend it right there. Whose meaning of money is being most met in this situation?

CHANGING VIEWS TOWARD MONEY

If a person does not see his personal world as being able to be transformed, it will undoubtedly stay the same. Fear of change, about money matters or any other arena in your life, manifests itself in the maintenance of rigid and frozen perceptions. However, despite these attitudes of limitation, human beings have the potential to make new discoveries that affect their perceptual awareness of the Universe and bring on growth of the psyche.

As Dr. James W. Woodard, a sociologist from Temple University, observed, "The historic answer of most groups to the problem of called-for change has been to buttress the status quo still further against the very changes called for—against the chaos and unpredictability occasioned by the inevitable transition period."[81] This quote from Dr. Woodard in the 1930s remains quite accurate even today, especially when it comes to lifestyle and economic changes in a person's life. It is much harder to create than it is to critique and destroy: just visualize the time one child takes building a sand castle and how swiftly another child can smash it down.

Changes in your perceived self change how you utilize resources. How do you spend your money if you believe in yourself? Where does your money go when you lack faith in yourself? Some maintain that if you are a student, you must take on considerable debt for a higher education. This expense can discourage you from pursuing your dreams and achieving self-actualization. Yet, after completing your education, you are generally capable of increasing your income, as well as accepting many new opportunities and possibilities for change in your life associated with reorganization of your perceived Universe. These possibilities bring an increased degree of adequacy. The good news is that once knowledge has expanded your perceptual awareness, it is difficult to restrict your perceived Universe in the same old ways.

Changes in how you perceive reality change how you obtain resources. An elderly gentleman, a former physical laborer, observed a graduate student client of mine reading, writing, and using his computer, and he asked that student, "When are you looking for employment?" He was seeing a Universe where employed people go to an office or work site and trying to fit the student's life into that box. He did not realize that the student was earning money at that moment over the Internet with his writing and computer skills. The elderly gentleman's past experiences blocked his ability to see new perspectives of experience potentially visible to him.

A future therapist takes on the expense of psychotherapy for herself and additional studies to enhance her knowledge and ability to work with future clients, while another student closes off those possibilities with the excuse, "I can't go to therapy. It is too expensive." Can anyone who has never undergone therapy really expect to work just as effectively with clients as the person who has already been through personal therapy?

Some individuals might expect to get away with little preparation or minimal service, yet charge the most dollars. One example is a landlord who fails to make needed repairs but doesn't forget to cash the monthly rent check. There is a huckster mentality at work in people who have not developed their skills or recognized their personal power. Investing in one's self is a commitment that requires us to step away from consensus or limited thinking. And investing in yourself comes with rewards; your finances can become increasingly healthy, along with your sense of adequacy when you dare to respect yourself, challenge yourself, and act accordingly.

DEFLECTING MESSAGES IN ADVERTISEMENTS

Advertisers control and alter our perceived Universe. Today's supposed truth may be falsely created—determined by those who have the most money to promote a particular point of view or pay for research and other marketing tools. An example would be the flood of advertising and research reports on various drugs to cure peoples' ailments, which overpowers any information about individuals using other methods of effectively healing, because alternative medical practitioners often lack resources, such as time and money, to promulgate their work. How persons attain and use money symbolizes who they truly are as human beings and how they relate to others in their world. The language in most advertisements tends to narrow the boundaries of understanding, excluding other options in order to highlight a given product or point of view and to stamp out opposing voices. This is an imposed differentiation. Dr. William Sargant, a British psychiatrist, emphasized that the target is the ordinary consumer, who is influenced to spend his or her meager income to provide the seller, ultimately, with massive economic power. This power is unfortunately too often used toward marketing campaigns that are in effect a form of hypnotic suggestion.[82]

Advertising and all other forms of creative media communication have the potential to increase your tendency to perceive threat. In techniques of brainwashing and mind control, there is an attempt made to increase the perceived threat in order to reorganize or diminish your understanding of your world and your definition of self. Feeling unsafe or threatened evokes strong emotions such as fear, anger, guilt, contempt, anxiety, jealousy, love, and excitement. Over time these emotions narrow your perceived Universe and create mental, emotional, and bodily exhaustion. Intense emotional arousal narrows your attention. In turn, narrowed attention restricts your perceptual possibilities and your ability to more fully apprehend your world. Fatigue also increases the likelihood that your perceptions can be distorted and exacerbates the potential for external forces to influence you. (These, by the way, are perfect conditions to set the stage for addiction—whether addiction to spending, food, substances, sex, or obsessive thoughts.)

Most money problems and their symptoms involve some form of hypnotic experience. Big business advertising targets your fears by bringing present perceptions of money into higher levels of awareness, in hopes that you respond in a way that ends up being financially beneficial for business, rather than for you, the target. Motivated by your need for adequacy, you attempt to use your money in the most effective manner. In cases where your perceptions are distorted, you might act in a way that corresponds to what seems to be real to you at the time, but might not necessarily be the most effective approach you could take—and would differ if you had a more accurate view of the world. Common impulsive behaviors involving money include:

- Shopping and purchasing items that the buyer doesn't really need
- Spending money on an expensive beauty treatment or a top-of-the-line power tool to combat depression and feel better
- Taking a trip to a gambling casino in the belief that it will lift one's spirits (among the most destructive compulsive decisions—as the odds are against such an excursion improving one's finances or resolving depression)

Just think about how you learned the word "dog" and how the word was paired with a picture of a dog. This explanation is beginning to sound more like hypnosis with every word you read, is it not? As explained by Stephen Jay Gould, an American paleontologist, evolutionary biologist, and historian of science who taught at Harvard University, "suggestions embedded in advertisements for particular products rouse uncontrollable associations that become linked to those products in an individual's field of awareness."[83] It appears that advertisers are increasingly using psychology in their work to impact you, and it is known that advertising firms have psychologists in their employ. In everyday life, images are flashed before your eyes that evoke love, loyalty, and trust while you are asked to purchase a product or endorse a candidate. For example, heavenly and celestial images are evoked intentionally in the symbolic language of advertising to access what Carl Jung calls the collective unconscious—the universality of a common human perceptual awareness experienced by all people in all cultures. These images are paired with products such as clothing or automobiles, and after stirring your deeper sense of being human, connect this experience with specific consumer behavior. This wealth of undifferentiated material and its influences are perceptually experienced at low levels of awareness. They subtly suggest how sexy and popular you will be if you smoke a certain brand of cigarette, drink a particular beer, buy a certain car, or wear designer clothing or sneakers.

You experience advertising and similar suggestions from others every day of your life. If you remain unaware, these suggestions can begin to form a personal reality. The real danger in everyday life is when so many things are happening around you that some suggestions from others go unnoticed and pass into your consciousness. For example, in one test of subliminal advertising, a ridiculous scene amuses the viewer, causing laughter about an absurdity, while the product message passes unnoticed into the viewer's mind.

Author Christina Merrill pinpointed an attempt of an advertiser to influence by using an actual hypnotist to sell Dewar's Scotch. This company's hypnotist used age regression on a group of adults to uncover their first experiences of drinking scotch, which happened at an earlier time in their lives. By use of this technique, the company ended up developing advertisements that connected the product with risk-taking images.[84] The hope was to associate drinking their product with memories of pleasant, exciting, and social times, perhaps in college or early in a career.

In a totally different (and more typical) setting, where a hypnotist is not trying to help sell a product but is working with a client and has that client's interests at heart, some individuals have successfully stopped drinking alcohol or quit smoking through hypnosis. Those individuals use hypnosis not only to battle their own tendencies, but to fight off advertisers' attempts to manipulate them.

When perception and suggestion merge in harmony, one enhances the other. For instance, an alcoholic client of mine used perceptual hypnosis to remove suggestions that his ability to drink large quantities of alcohol proved he was a real man—an idea that could have been implanted in his mind early in life. Hypnosis helped him see that the idea was a suggestion he'd absorbed, but did not reflect the real Universe—or who he was. As perceptual hypnosis brings both hypnotic experience and the use of suggestion in advertising into higher levels of awareness, it creates the opportunity to reorganize your perceived Universe by applying a newly learned perspective.

Purchasing behavior is like a post-hypnotic suggestion being carried out after hypnosis, a spontaneous reappearance of a past organization of a perceived Universe. How is this simple technique being utilized to exert even greater influence on individuals and groups? Another commercial that illustrates the same principle, but is more subtle, starts off with small white circles on a black background that slowly increase in size until the viewers feel like they are moving through a tunnel. At the end of this advertisement, a red circle with numbers signifying that product is printed in the center, which then changes into a rectangle with the product name. This is a more subtle approach, but hypnosis just the same. More sophisticated advertisements can have far more subtle effects that result in greater consequences for those they influence.

THE HYPNOTIC PROCESS IN BIG BUSINESS AND THE MEDIA

Mass media is another external influence that needs conscious attention so that one isn't unwittingly victimized by its designs and has many implications for perceptual awareness and hypnotic experience in your life. The media often manipulate and control your perceptions at low levels of awareness when you are unsuspecting. As Erich Fromm, a German psychologist, pointed out, the effects of advertising are comparable to the effects of an opiate or instantaneous hypnosis.[85]

BIG BUSINESS

Big business advertising has produced results using suggestion and creating distorted perceptions while developing, researching, and exploiting hypnotic experience and attempting to manipulate perceptual processes in many individuals.

As Dr. William Wesley Cook, a physician, put it back in 1927:

They will repeat over and over again, in a loud and tiresome voice, the good qualities of their wares, and by looks and gestures rivet attention upon themselves, and finally succeed in securing a high price for a poor article from a customer who will acknowledge afterward that he was completely taken in.[86]

Carl Sextus, who was a Danish hypnotist described a similar situation that is still relevant today:

Supposing two businessmen come together. One, without the other having the least idea of it, is studying the weak points of his associate. The stronger and more intelligent of the two will, after a while, bring the other to look upon the subject as he desires, and finally to submit to his wishes. This then is suggestion with hypnotic influence, though the person is perfectly awake. The person upon whom the influence is brought to bear imagines himself to be possessing all his senses, while at the same time he is bound to submit to the influence of the other. As a result of this kind of suggestion many otherwise shrewd businessmen are frequently led to enter upon business enterprises which they, under other conditions, when exactly the same offers were made by the same people, refused to accept or consider; because they then followed their own particular interest; and hence they did not commit any folly to regret later on. As soon as the weaker party is out of the sight of the stronger, the former perceives his blunder, but, alas, too late.[87]

You can see how this influence occurs in life if you think of commercials as representing shrewd businessmen. For instance, after viewing or hearing a commercial a few times, your mind may recall an entire experience of this commercial with just a flash of a segment. You may perceive these brief snippets as you flip through channels, or see a condensed version of the commercial being shown for such popular events as the Super Bowl, the Miss America Pageant, or the Olympics. Because of prior exposure, your mind recalls this entire commercial while the advertiser pays less for the more expensive time spots at these major events.

Do these suggestions maintain or enhance your sense of self? Aspects of your perceived self may be amazingly unknown to you, as you carry the advertisers' suggestions out at a later time. Other hypnotic tricks used in an advertisement might include changes in color and lighting, quick switches of images, changes in scenes and locations, and an increase in the volume of voices, noises, and other sounds. These effects can be deployed to alter your perceptual awareness, much the way hypnotists in the movies sometimes use a swinging watch to change your focus or attention. Simply put, as you change what you differentiate, you alter your experience.

Particular commercials target particular types of people who have a need for adequacy. A television commercial presents a hair color product using the scene of a wedding with a statement, ". . . even if your marriage doesn't last, your color will!" On what group of people is this commercial suggestion focused? After an image is presented, it must connect with someone's need for adequacy to be effective. People not concerned about their appearance will not place this hair coloring commercial in higher levels of awareness. People who experience issues in their marriages might place this commercial in a midrange level of awareness, still at a relatively low level, but at a somewhat higher level of awareness than the former group because of the attempt to connect improving your marriage with improving your appearance.

In *Basic Statistical Analysis*, Dr. Richard Sprinthall, former chairman of the psychology department at American International College in Springfield, Massachusetts, pointed out perceptual distortions in a Volvo commercial where a gigantic pickup truck called "Big Bear" crushed the tops of a row of automobiles—all of them, of course, except a Volvo. In reality, this Volvo was reinforced with extra steel columns, while the structural supports of all the other cars were removed.[88] In a different type of example, a woman told me that, as an employee of a major department store, she witnessed ". . . that just prior to any sale, the store always increased their regular prices of the items going on sale, so that the sale price was in relationship to this [newer] prior regular price." This type of ploy is a quite effective distortion of perception, creating a change in behavior on the part of a consumer. Recently, I observed this phenomenon in a department store that had a going-out-of-business sale. The DVDs were 50 percent off the regular price, but they were still higher than another store's regular price for the same DVD.

An orthodontist shared with me that some dental companies advertise extracting three wisdom teeth at a given price with the fourth wisdom tooth free. The funny thing is, the price is no different than the regular price of having all four wisdom teeth removed by the average dentist. People respond favorably to the perceived benefit of such an advertisement, even though there is no discount in reality.

Your perceptions and personal meanings are constantly being shaped through external influences. You often do not accurately see what is before you. This way of "seeing" occurs, for example, when you are mistreated by a large organization that employs you or provides services to others.

When discussing corporate violence, Dr. John Monahan, psychologist and professor of law, and Dr. Raymond Novaco, professor of psychology and social behavior at Indiana University, explained such mistreatment and defined corporate violence as acts producing dangers of physical harm to consumers, employees, or other persons as a consequence of deliberate decision making or culpable negligence by corporate executives.[89]

Once a perceived threat from an organization or corporation comes into higher levels of awareness, you tend to place this threat back in lower levels of awareness and allow it to affect you from there. Instead, you could examine it accurately and act accordingly.

An example of the type of corporate violence Dr. Novaco refers to was perpetrated at a psychiatric institution and a counseling center by administrators and other staff who controlled access to services and evaluated treatment benefits from a monetary gain perspective only, while at the same time allowing aggression toward individuals whose insurances paid less to go unchecked. Such aggressions include referring out to other providers, refusing to take the insurance, increasing prices due to increased auxiliary staff driven by needs for higher profits, etc. Occurrences of this type of violence must not remain hidden. Examining the threat as soon as it is perceived is critically important in such cases.

I'm reminded of the comment by a behavioral specialist and supervisor at a middle school who stated upon observing a twelve-year-old girl who lived in a low-income housing project with her mentally ill mother: "How can she have a new coat?" This woman, with a good salary, husband, and house, begrudged this poor girl having a coat her grandparents bought her for Christmas. The woman demonstrated an inability to identify with the child. Apparently, her own adequacy was threatened by the girl's having a new coat.

THE MEDIA

While there are those in the media who attempt to distort perception, there are others who provide viewpoints that enhance changing and expanding perceptions. For example, television shows such as the *X-Files* in the 1990s, and *The 4400* in the 2000s, with themes of paranormal phenomena, and the movie *The Matrix* portray how common perceptions shared by the majority of people may be deceptive in their essence. Such productions demonstrate the significance of looking beyond the surface of things and exploring the hidden meanings that often go undetected. After all, what would your reality be if you found that alien beings existed that were far different and more advanced than your civilization? Seeing the possibilities in these shows keeps you open to new ideas, allowing your perceived Universe to expand.

In some cases an actor can provide an alternative viewpoint, such as when Steven Seagal, an actor and environmental activist, spoke out at the end of the movie *On Deadly Ground* against corruption of big business and the poisoning of the earth, They influence the media so they can control our minds; they've made it a crime for us to speak out and if we do, we are called conspiracy nuts . . . they have no cure for the world they destroy, only for the money they make in the process.

Dr. William Sargant likewise brought attention to the true reason that lobotomy remained an acceptable treatment for so long. When discussing brain surgery on mentally ill persons, he delivered a message similar to Seagal's with regard to people who don't conform in society:

> [T]he success of leucotomy [lobotomy] is a reminder of the uselessness of the merely rational approach to many patients suffering from fixed ideas; and of the consequent unhappy recourse, throughout history, to lunatic asylums, prisons, concentration camps, gallows, or the stake as a means of removing from society all individuals who cannot otherwise be made to accept the beliefs accepted by the more ordinary and suggestible majority.[90]

As you saw earlier, advertising is an external influence that functions through creating distorted perceptions. It links words with images, emotions, bodily awareness, and other aspects of your experience that remain at very low levels of awareness. It associates and mirrors your needs and desires with a particular product or service through as many aspects of your perceived Universe as can be stimulated.

A simple example would be an advertisement with your favorite song playing in the background, a song with lyrics about a loving relationship. This may stimulate you to recall an image of your grandfather in his favorite chair, your former lover, or a close friend from your childhood, and positive experiences you had with these individuals. As a result, while hearing this song, you may remember or re-experience your bodily awareness from that earlier time, or perceive external aspects of your world that the song brings to mind—your emotions, your thoughts, pleasant smells, and many other positive aspects of your perceived world both then and now. You also may remember or call back into awareness experiences from early in your life that cannot be put into words. These are sometimes called preverbal experiences—experiences that you had as a child prior to an understanding of language. The possible effect on this area of your mind is where the most danger in advertising lies.

Naturally or intentionally, advertising affects preverbal aspects of experience, often at very low levels of awareness. In *The Clam Plate Orgy*, Dr. Wilson Bryan Key, who attained a PhD in communications at Denver University, pointed out that sexual organs are implanted in ads to seduce the consumer to purchase particular products.[91] These images, placed at low levels of awareness, may enhance purchase

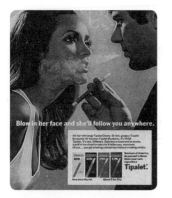

Blow in her face and she'll follow you anywhere.

of a product by altering your differentiations and speaking to your need for adequacy.

Television isn't the only medium used to hypnotize people. At the turn of the twentieth century, when Jay Walter Thompson became vice-president of the largest advertising agency in New York City, he engaged J.

Tipalet cigarette advertisement, c. 1960. Distortion of reality.

B. Watson, founder of behaviorism in the 1920s, to use psychological knowledge to change women's perceptions of smoking by creating successful magazine ads. These ads changed the impression widely held at the time that only harlots smoked cigarettes. An artful manipulation of smoking showed an overweight woman lying on a couch with a pack of Lucky Strikes and chocolates on a coffee table. The message was to reach for a cigarette and not a sweet. Another layout showed an image of a virginal or innocent woman as smoke drifts toward her with the message: "blow a little my way."[92] On page 113 is an example of an old advertisement about smoking tobacco.

What a change from today's view of smoking! What other techniques and methods of the modern era of television commercials and Internet advertising are being used to manipulate people's perception and affect behavior?

Not only commercials but news events as well, alter people's awareness. How many people, engrossed in their busy daily lives, are healthy and functioning well until they hear on their radios or watch a news report on television about a flu epidemic? Soon they, too, may have the flu. Dr. G. H. Estabrooks, a prominent psychologist, stated back in 1957 in his book *Hypnotism*, "So we do have hypnotism of a very effective type over the radio and television, but it bears another label."[93]

During Super Bowl XXX in 1996, a Pepsi commercial portrayed someone pouring Pepsi into a fish tank, followed by the fish in the tank responding with a number of aquatic tricks. Within days children throughout the country began pouring Pepsi into their fish tanks to see if their fish would do similar tricks. In this instance, the power of suggestion from television advertising cannot be disputed. No wonder Dr. Stephen Jay Gould asserted that the psychophysiological effects of watching a commercial should be compared to the effects of being hypnotized.[94] Some research suggests that watching television induces the alpha state associated with hypnosis and meditative states and enhances suggestibility. Remembering that original event was the essence of suggestion to those children and had more power than a command to execute a similar act could have had. The children identified with the person in the commercial.

Current perceptions can be reorganized to alter perception of past behaviors. A number of former hypnosis clients, who have stopped smoking cigarettes after a group hypnosis session, began to smoke again after watching movies that glamorized smoking, such as the aptly titled *Smoke*. Some of these clients returned for further sessions of hypnosis, stating that these films had interfered with their progress.

S. L. Hwang, a staff reporter at the *Wall Street Journal*, pointed out that "smoxploitation" movies like *Paula*, *Smoky Kisses*, *The Two Sides of April*, and *Selena*, all glamorize and eroticize smoking.[95] Despite today's unpopular perceptions of smoking that are turning the habit into a fetish and taboo, clearly images that glamorize smoking produce perceptions that do have an impact on behavior and must be countered with hypnotic perceptions of nonsmoking experiences. These external influences are well realized by clients, who report that smoking their first cigarette caused unpleasant nausea, vomiting, coughing, and dizziness—effects that were overcome by peer pressure from their friends.

MEDIA PORTRAYAL OF HYPNOSIS

The media sometimes sensationalizes experiences of hypnosis. In a documentary television show *Hard Copy*, a production of Paramount Pictures, a hypnotic dog named Oscar was portrayed in a December 1995 segment. In the program a number of volunteers, who had stared into Oscar's eyes, were shown sitting on a bench and then slumping over and falling uncontrollably asleep on the floor, one at a time, until a heap of people resulted. The message of this allegedly informative news piece was that even a dog can hypnotize you and make you fall asleep. The black Labrador retriever in the film, in actuality, was a prop for entertainment hypnotist Hugh Lennon. Such a prop is no different from a watch or a spot on the wall, simply used as a means to get a person to relax so hypnosis may begin!

Some television portrayals of hypnosis leave viewers feeling that the process is equivalent to a victim falling under the spell of a vampire in an old-fashioned Dracula movie. These portrayals almost always contain a situation involving lost love or a victim who blocked out a threatening episode. The hypnotist typically aids in memory recall of a highly sensational and stressful life circumstance, such as a crime, an alien abduction, a rape while under anesthesia, or a similar traumatic incident someone may have chosen to forget. The techniques used during these television episodes are as magically brief and based on misinformation as are the silly and theatrical portrayals of hypnosis.

An individual can re-experience a traumatic event in everyday life when exposed to cues that symbolize or resemble the original event. This happens with veterans as well as abused children. The authors of the *DSM-IV Casebook* discussed a case of post traumatic stress disorder in which a fire in a dress factory triggered memories of 1943 Auschwitz in a sixty-seven-year-old woman who was only seventeen years old at the time.[96] Dr. Robert L. Spitzer and colleagues, editors of the *DMS-IV*, were unable to understand why the woman remembered the experience, stating, "Why such a relatively minor event could trigger such an extreme response after so many years is a mystery."[97] Yet having any current real or imagined experience or even seeing a movie or television show with details that have similarities to those in a past organization of a person's perceived Universe or self can evoke memories of past threatening experience by bringing that event into higher levels of awareness. The power of media cannot be underestimated. This used to happen to an associate of mine whenever she watched a television program that had a trial taking place. "I couldn't watch *Law and Order* for years and years. I was in the "audience" for a real murder trial and watched the state's attorney defend the man who killed my grandmother. It was horrible, and I can say I had much trouble getting over it. I still have some trouble, but not like I used to. I actually replaced the memory of the trial with a funny law show that came on a few years ago staring Cathy Bates—I forget the name. After that, I seemed to be okay. I still cringe just a bit though, but I'm finally getting over it." The media does indeed have power, sometimes unintended.

The media has also presented accurate and educational programs on hypnosis. Documentaries, brief news stories, and accounts of those bringing back seemingly impossible memories through hypnosis have also been aired on television, such as individuals recalling information on a WW II ship at Pearl Harbor and remembering accurate information that led to finding money and weapons under a house in the South where slaves were smuggled north for freedom.

Some programs have demonstrated an increasing use of hypnosis for solving numerous personal problems, such as weight loss or smoking cessation. The programs that have demonstrated the benefits of hypnosis have done so in a responsible and accurate manner, concluding that if you really wish to understand hypnosis, you should experience hypnosis for yourself. In this chapter you have seen how many types of external influences have gone unchecked and unexamined in life. Now that you are aware of some of the ways that you might be influenced in everyday life and some of the perceptual options to counter such influence, it should be clear how enhanced perceptual awareness makes for wiser consumer choices. Once you begin to understand how perceptual awareness is formed and changed in everyday life, it becomes more difficult for outside forces to influence you without your being aware of it. Society and helping professionals must remember to address external influences that are contributing to clients' psychological suffering in the process of helping individuals adapt to the world—and to those very external influences.

PERCEPTUAL POINTS

- Through awareness of perceptual dynamics, you can protect yourself from external influences that don't have your best interests in mind.
- The way you relate to money mirrors your relationships to others.
- Advertisers know your mind recalls an entire experience with just a flash of a segment of that experience.

PERCEPTUAL EXERCISE

Find some outdated suggestions from your past that led to beliefs. When looking for possible suggestions to change, answer this question: Where do you see the Earth as flat in your life? You might have thoughts such as:

1. I can't lose weight.
2. I have no time to exercise.
3. I'm not as smart as my friend [parent, sibling, spouse].
4. I will never be promoted.

Revise those suggestions to change them into new positive perceptions, like these:

1. See yourself having lost weight.
2. See yourself exercising.
3. See yourself as smart as your friend [parent, sibling, spouse].
4. See yourself getting promoted.

Spend time visualizing these suggestions every day and notice the results.

CHAPTER NINE

THE RELATIONSHIP OF HYPNOSIS TO RELIGION AND SPIRITUALITY

"In bringing a spiritual dimension to the context of psychotherapy, we are not referring to the application of religious dogma, but to a type of knowing which transcends the intellect and has sometimes been referred to as the magical or mystical."[98]

— *L. J. Phillips and J. W. Osborne*

One topic that always comes up when someone is attempting to understand hypnosis is its relationship to religion and spirituality in one's life. There are many aspects of perceptual hypnosis that are relevant to discussion of this topic. The Christian viewpoint of hypnosis is thoroughly explored in this chapter as are other religious viewpoints.

CHRISTIANITY AND HYPNOSIS

Hypnotic experience can expand perceptual awareness of one's spirituality and thereby assist one in discovering hidden potential in this realm. Religious leaders and other professionals demonstrate both confusion and misunderstanding when it comes to these phenomena of hypnosis. Ancient wisdom, such as is contained in the Bible and expressed in the life of Jesus, speaks on behalf of awakening hidden potential. Religion and spirituality appear to be quite different concepts that can be compatible with or in conflict with your perceived Universe and self.

The distinction between religious and spiritual is analogous to the difference between quantitative and qualitative. Religious often refers to an objective organized dogma and ritual behavior in groups, organized with a hierarchy of power and tied strongly to the physical world. Spiritual is a subjective individual experience in the Universe (associated with God or a higher power) that usually transcends time and space and emphasizes individuality. Spiritual would be seen as ethical while religious would be moral. More and more of my clinical and research clients are identifying themselves as spiritual rather than religious.

Both religious and spiritual experiences reported throughout history have demonstrated that humans are far more than just physical beings separate from each other and from the Universe. Instead, those experiences provide synchronistic evidence that individual perceptual awareness and personal meanings affect human thoughts, feelings, and behavior.

For example, at the time of Abraham Lincoln's assassination, General Grant and his wife, Julia, were supposed to join the president and his wife at Ford Theater. Julia Grant "felt a great sense of urgency that she, her husband, and their child should leave Washington and return to their home in New Jersey." After Julia repeatedly pleaded with her husband on several different occasions, the Grants chose to return home rather than go to Ford's theater that night. Not only were they to be sitting next to President Lincoln, but General Grant, a future president of the United States, was also an intended victim of John Wilkes Booth.[99]

Another example was a precognition of the Arab surprise attack on the Day of Atonement, 1973, by an English housewife. While meditating she had a vision about the Arab attack two weeks before the actual event took place and then sent a letter to Golda Meir, the Israeli Prime Minister, four days before the incident happened. The postmark on the letter bears evidence to the spiritual event. The woman had no personal ties and little knowledge of Israel, yet her description of the local government and the surprise attack were in sufficient detail to verify the vision.[100] This precognition allowed Israel to prevent a terrorist attack.

Validation of most spiritual experiences involves the synchronicity of a subjective inner experience with a subsequent physical event. I have experienced several events in my own life. While beginning to hypnotize a subject for phenomenological research, I repetitively had the thought to say to him that he knows he can open his eyes, but he doesn't need to do that at this moment. I did not verbally express this inner thought but kept it to myself so as not to interfere with his hypnotic experience. Upon interviewing him after the hypnosis session, he stated he repeatedly had the thought he could open his eyes at the beginning of being hypnotized and this had interfered with his relaxing until he stopped thinking about it.

Another case was when I was contemplating a research example of a spiritual experience that occurred in Nashua, New Hampshire, in the 1970s, where a single mother of three daughters had left an appointment and was involved in an accident. While sitting in her damaged car she perceived herself taken through the window of a car by a man in all white (even though her large body would not have fit through the window) just prior to another vehicle totaling her car in a way that would have most likely taken her life.[101] While reading a biography on the life of Padre Pio, I came across a story in his book where a pharmacist overseas, whose car plunged into the Adriatic Sea, was rescued by someone in a great light who took him through his car window, even though his large body should have made such an act impossible.[102] These stories were so similar I was amazed I had even stumbled across it.

When you take into account that Richard Wain, a Kent SE London Support Network Coordinator for the British Institute of Hypnotherapy, asserted that hypnotic experience has been described in the Bible,[103] there is no reason that religion, spirituality, and hypnosis cannot enhance each other. The real battle is whether professional hypnotists, religious leaders, and spiritual teachers are attempting to enhance individual realities and personal meanings or to control and define perceptions and personal meanings for others.

Few individuals realize that the Bible considers spiritual abilities to be spiritual gifts given individually to different human beings so that they can better help others. In the Old King James Bible, St. Paul told the Corinthians in Chapter 12:

> Now concerning spiritual gifts, brethren, I would not have you ignorant [Verse 1] . . . Now there are diversities of gifts,
> but the same Spirit [Verse 4]. . . And there are diversities of operations,
> but it is the same God which worketh all in all [Verse 6]. . .
> For to one is given by the Spirit the word of wisdom;
> to another the word of knowledge by the same Spirit;
> To another faith by the same Spirit;
> to another the gifts of healing by the same Spirit;
> To another the working of miracles;
> to another prophecy;
> to another discerning of spirits;
> to another diverse kinds of tongues;
> to another the interpretation of tongues;
> But all these worketh that one and the selfsame
> Spirit, dividing to every man severally as he will. [Verse 8-11][104]
> (Scripture taken from the KJHB—Giant Print. Copyright © 1976 by
> Thomas Nelson
> Used by permission. All rights reserved.)

The oneness principle expressed by Jesus explains that when we hurt another, we hurt ourselves. Despite the fact that this explanation occurs in the New Testament as a teaching of Jesus, some go back to the Old Testament and refute the support of hypnosis with alternative quotes that condemn individuals with special gifts and advocate stoning them to death, out of fear of the unknown and ignorance. Many are told to only listen to "the Lord's Word" in the Bible, yet there are those who will conveniently interpret the Word for you, labeling hypnosis as, for example, evil or antireligious. There are numerous ways of interpreting the information from the Bible that a religious person hears in everyday conversations with other religious people. Who rightfully knows the true words of God that might be in the Bible, after so many translations and so much subsequent editing? A dear friend and Catholic Priest once told me that the Old King James Version of the Bible is the closest English translation to the original work. As close as that is, however, even King James decided some passages should not be published. The bottom line spiritually is nicely put by Friar Giles, a close associate of St. Francis of Assisi, who stated: "Everything that a man doeth, good or evil, he doeth it to himself."[105]

A religious person once told me that ". . . the Bible is against hypnosis," yet Christian principles are nowhere violated through the use of hypnosis. The Catholic Church has approved the use of hypnosis. Some fundamentalists, Seventh Day Adventists, and Christian Scientists continue to utilize the natural healing abilities of hypnosis, while remaining uneducated and misguided about how hypnosis is actually manifested in everyday lives.

Several spiritual leaders experienced hypnosis prior to their religious contributions to society. Mary Baker Eddy, who founded Christian Science Church, suffered from spinal weakness and spasmodic seizures that Dr. Phineas Parkhurst Quimby, inventor and mesmerist, healed with hypnosis in 1862. She published a letter in the *Portland Courier* praising his healing abilities. A traveling hypnotist discovered the abilities of the Christian healer Edgar Cayce. Mother Ann, founder of the Shakers, had an incidence of religious ecstasy where blood spontaneously appeared through the pores of her skin.[106]

In light of these reports of spiritual people having heightened perceptual awareness, why does the goal of awakening people to their own innate abilities meet with such opposition from some Christians? Alexander Docker, PhD, former president of the American Board of Hypnotherapy, offers a possible answer that explains the objections coming from the fundamentalist branches of Christianity:

> Fundamentalism, of any religious persuasion, is simply the expression of a need to control and organize the spiritual experience of all peoples in accordance with a [single] person's own narrow view of reality.[107]

This type of fundamental extremism in any religion tends to drive people away from the spiritual abilities that they might possess and deters them from encountering spiritually oriented healing techniques, including hypnosis.

Psychotherapy conducted within a spiritual or paranormal framework is a very different form of therapy than many conventionally trained psychotherapists attempt. One reason it is so different is that the spiritual individual's boundaries of the sense of self might be much more expanded than in conventional thought, transcending some time and space limitations. The spiritual person might know at some level of awareness how grandma feels in California even if he or she is in New Hampshire. Some persons have a much deeper relationship with the Universe than others.

In a spiritual world, there may be consequences for actions that go beyond simple cause and effect. Being ruthless on the job or intelligent enough to seduce someone into handing over resources or money may affect your child or relatives years later, even after your death. A story from science fiction that could very well be true might be that of a psychiatrist who medicates a patient for having hallucinations and communications with her grandmother, yet later dies and encounters the grandmother of his patient, who actually *was* communicating with his patient, and he learns he was interfering with their communications.

The point is that, phenomenologically, you try to have an open mind to experiences that you may or may not have had yourself, interfering only when those experiences might truly harm an individual's life. There are many examples of people attempting to expand their beliefs and perceptions of experiences that are far more complex than anticipated.

A mental health counselor responded this way, "I'm going to start a group for teenage girls who see ghosts; there are a lot of them around here." When I asked her how she would handle it when one of those girls psychically tuned in on her inner experience, she stated: "They can't really do that." The counselor professed to have the ability to determine whether others perceive another dimension of experience or not. The work of helping professionals should never exploit another as the counselor spoke of doing, but rather enhance their lives.

A spiritually-oriented therapist must always keep in mind that your spirituality is a way of viewing the personal meaning of your life or understandings. Although professionals don't need to be experts in every type of religion or spiritual experience, it is crucial that they respect others' beliefs and points of view.

It is my opinion that only persons at the extremes are leery of a union between science and spirituality. At one end are the zealots or fanatics who have twisted religion or spirituality to suit their own very narrow needs. At the other end are scientists who refuse to accept any spiritual phenomena even exist because those phenomena don't fit a restricted ideology, specific training, or expertise of their field of science. Paul Tillich's views on the spiritual fanatic fit very well here:

> Fanaticism is the correlate to spiritual self-surrender: it shows the anxiety, which it was supposed to conquer, by attacking with disproportionate violence those who disagree and who demonstrate by their disagreement elements in the spiritual life of the fanatic which he must suppress in himself. Because he must suppress them in himself he must suppress them in others. His anxiety forces him to persecute dissenters. The weakness of the fanatic is that those whom he fights have a secret hold upon him; and to this weakness he and his group finally succumb.[108]

In a way, Paul Tillich shows how others attempt to restrict your view of the Universe in order to maintain the validity of their own perceived Universes or realities. These people know that you and other people seek acknowledgment and recognition and often compare yourselves to others. Whether you are a fanatic or a scientist, you can hide a distorted perception in an intellectual viewpoint with a personal ideology. While reason and statistical probabilities can help people understand the positive aspects of individual differences and avoid suppressing them, expanding awareness helps you focus and achieve self-discovery and clarity first. Of the manipulators who would restrict your Universe, Dr. Eugene Taylor stated: "The great lesson of history is to keep the power of life and death away from the kind of mind, the mind that sees things in the light of evil and dread and mistrust, rather than in that of hope."[109]

Would-be manipulators have to understand that they cannot gain personal self-growth or change that leads to fulfilling their dreams and hidden potential unless they can expand their own Universes. They can do this by extending their perceptions and personal meanings. This expansion does not involve using their critical eye to compare and criticize others who are different. Rather it involves embracing others, and learning from their differences, using interactions with others as an opportunity to expand their own knowledge about love, acceptance, and understanding. Such an expansion of the entire Universe can lead to a win-win situation in which everyone grows.

JESUS WARNED AGAINST BEING UNAWARE

In the Bible, Jesus would not take up the cause of the zealot, who often used hypnotic-like techniques to get unsuspecting individuals or, worse, wounded individuals, to accept his ideas uncritically. Jesus encouraged people, as does perceptual hypnosis, to perceive life and the world as accurately as possible—a goal that people should embrace. Jesus warned against distorted perceiving as he is quoted in Matthew 7:3–5 as stating:

> And why beholdest thou the mote that is in thy brother's eye,
> but considerest not the beam that is in thine own eye?
> Or how wilt thou say to thy brother, Let me pull out the mote out of thine eye,
> and, behold, a beam is in thine own eye? Thou hypocrite, first cast out the beam out of thine own eye, and then shalt thou see clearly to cast out the mote out of thy brother's eye.[110]

More simply stated: You must examine yourself before criticizing someone else. Self-examination in the profession of spiritually oriented therapy is an essential aspect of helping others. It is also the only path to self-growth. Once you think you already have the answers and believe these answers are unchanging, you have lost the chance to find the truth of life.

STIGMATA—KEY TO UNDERSTANDING HYPNOTIC PHENOMENA

An interesting spiritual phenomenon that may help shed light on the powers of hypnosis and the mind and brings the physical, psychological, and spiritual aspects of human experience together is the stigmata. Stigmata are visible manifestations of wounds similar to those suffered by Jesus Christ in the crucifixion that are found in some human beings. These people (known as stigmatics) have a highly developed sense of empathy and so identify with another person's experience—such as the sufferings of Jesus Christ as recorded in the Bible and reproduced in art throughout the world—that they subjectively become one with that experience. (In a similar fashion, healers have to be cautious about absorbing the illness of those they heal.)

Hypnosis has already demonstrated that your mental images and internal experience can make changes in your physical body. For example, hypnotists have produced changes in blood pressure, controlled bleeding, enlarged breasts, removed warts, and reproduced welts and marks that were caused by past traumas. In response to years of studying past-life experiences, Dr. Jim Tucker, medical director of the Child and Family Psychiatry Clinic and associate professor of psychiatry and neurobehavioral sciences at the University of Virginia School of Medicine, authored *Life Before Life: A Scientific Investigation of Children's Memories of Previous Lives*, which presents over forty years of reincarnation research at the Division of Perceptual Studies. Tucker, who suggests that birth marks may be a way of linking past and present lives, also suggests that a process similar to hypnosis is the mechanism that psychologically and spiritually produces these marks on the stigmatic's physical body.[111]

Prior to the physiological appearance of stigmata, individuals who manifest them often suffer severe illness or traumas that may include much internal subjective pain. Visible aspects of the stigmata have included (with no verifiable external physical cause):

- Open wounds bleeding from the palms, wrists, and feet;Welts on the shoulders (from carrying a cross) and on the back (from whips)
- Marks on the wrists (from cords)
- Wounds on the side (pierced by a spear)
- Marks on the forehead (crown of thorns)
- Bloody sweats and tears and visions of Mother Mary's perceptions of the crucifixion

Other aspects include: sweet smells of flowers and other scents; prior to the appearance of wounds, there are feelings of depression; feelings of weakness before wounds manifest; mismatch between the blood type of wound blood and a person's normal blood type. Those with stigmata experience ecstasy, visions, trance; have repulsion for food, have wounds that bleed on specific days; and have an absence of infection in these wounds. They get little if any sleep; undergo periods of prolonged prayer and meditation; experience guardian angels, hear voices, are demonically attacked, and experience paranormal abilities (healing, astral projection, levitation, psychokinesis, poltergeist activity, blood flowing against gravity, clairvoyance, a gift of prophecy, speaking with spirits).

Cases of stigmata have been verified in many ways, including by reputable eyewitnesses and by having the part of the body confined so that the person could not injure it. These controls help validate the experiences and suggest that other people have to accept that at least the stigmata manifested the power of the mind over the body.

Stigmatics are incredibly empathic and often experience strong emotions. The first known stigmatic was Saint Francis of Assisi (1181–1226) who received the stigmata after fasting for forty days and during prayer and meditation on the Feast of Exaltation of the Cross about September 14, 1224.

Bodily wounds can vary in form and location, depending on the individual stigmatic. For example, St. Francis had protrusions of flesh that formed the shapes of nails through his hands and feet. Open holes are seen in wounds on some stigmatic's hands; such was in the case of Padre Pio (1887–1968). Other stigmatics, who have wounds on their wrists rather than their palms, suggest cultural and perceptual influences affecting manifestations on their bodies, based on artwork in their possession depicting the time period in which they lived.

These sufferings, visible or invisible, can be factors that influence how those having hypnotic and paranormal experiences relate to their bodies, others, and the Universe. All such wounds are spontaneously experienced. Historically, genuine stigmatics had not necessarily sought publicity or material reward and were even embarrassed by the physical presence of their wounds. Phenomena of this sort are empathically considered in two alternative ways:

1. Bigger than people's egos (representative of unity in the Universe). Unity means empathic union with sources other than those familiar cause-and-effect relationships defined in the physical world. People are affected by sources beyond their clear awareness, reflecting the Taoist principle that people are all connected as one and the Native American connection between nature and the Earth.

2. Worthy of vengeful skepticism (representative of separation between aspects of the Universe). Separation is the "us versus them" syndrome of creating enemies and fighting over limited resources. People treat others as objects to be manipulated for their own selfish gain.

The phenomenon of the stigmata is mostly a Roman Catholic experience that has been most often found in fertile women of Europe (Belgium, England, France, Germany, Italy, Netherlands, Portugal, Spain, and Yugoslavia) who came from difficult and peasant backgrounds. Angela Della Pace (1610–62) was a child stigmatic at nine years old. While stigmata have been observed in the Italian Padre Pio, they have also been observed in a Protestant in Hamburg, Germany, and a ten-and-one-half-year-old African-American girl, who began to bleed in a California classroom. This last case is the only twentieth century recorded case of a child with stigmata that I know of, and she was examined and found by medical personnel to have no mental illness or other medical condition that would generate such wounds. Her family was highly religious (Baptist). She experienced voices that told her to pray with specific individuals. When she prayed with these individuals, they received healings that the voices foretold.[112] Some have claimed that both ancient and modern-day Islamics have suffered the same wounds that the Prophet Mohammed received in battle, a non-Christian experience that parallels the stigmata.

In relatively recent times (1800s), the stigmata experience spread to the Western hemisphere (Australia, the United States, and Canada). The stigmatic Louise Lateau (1850–83) was investigated by Dr. Ferdinand J.M. Lefebvre, a professor at Catholic University at Louvain, and several church officials.[113] Some stigmatics have been sainted.[114] More than 321 stigmatics have been identified. (See Appendix A for a partial list.)

Some believe that the wounds that appear as stigmata are created through the use of imagination with intense emotion. Others believe that stigmatics self-inflicted their wounds secretly when alone, or their wounds were "unconsciously" created under hypnosis or during somnambulism (sleep walking). Keep in mind that hypnosis is nothing other than natural human abilities in action; therefore, even if these wounds did occur under hypnosis, this does not invalidate stigmata. Rather, proving that an individual had these experiences under hypnosis validates them as genuine experiences of a human being in a particular perceived Universe. Stigmata would be a case of hypnotic suggestion affecting bodily functions that are not under voluntary control.

Hypnosis has been shown to have physical effects. Hypnosis has created blisters and other physical manifestations during an abreaction—demonstrating a link between human perceptual awareness and people's physical bodies. An abreaction is a reliving of a past event so as to release the emotional aspects connected to the event that continue at low levels of awareness to affect the person in the present. For example, consider the 1946 rope case: A thirty-five-year-old male participant who was hypnotized relived a past trauma when he was restrained from sleepwalking at a hospital. During hypnosis, indentations in his arms appeared and he bled from rope burns that had been inflicted in that past trauma. He was under strict observation during the study, to prevent fraud or self-injurious behavior. These wounds were photographed and presented in the journal *The Lancet*.[115]

Researchers have demonstrated how the memory of past experiences has created present physical changes in the body. Dr. Robert Moody, a psychiatrist at Woodside Hospital in London, England, cited bodily changes in several patients reliving past traumas, such as a thirty-five-year-old woman who recalled a childhood riding accident and re-experienced hemorrhages and bruising during her recollection.[116] Menzies demonstrated reduced skin temperature in participants who imagined past experiences of extreme cold.[117]

The fact that hypnosis has produced changes in the physical body is quite well documented and is a bridge to understanding the stigmata. Dr. Alfred Lechler, a Christian psychiatrist, created the stigmata with hypnosis in his client, Elizabeth K., generating marks on her forehead and bleeding as she focused upon Jesus's crown of thorns in the crucifixion and marks he received from scourging.[118, 119, 120]

Similar phenomena are psychogenic purpura—red and purple wound discoloration on the skin—spontaneous lesions that appear on a person's body in relation to the re-experience of a past trauma. Dr. J. E. Lifschutz, an American psychiatrist, presented a case of a forty-six-year-old female who bled anew from scars that her father had inflicted when she was thirteen years old whenever she was intensely emotional or when visiting him. Another case of psychogenic purpura occurred in a hypnotized subject who manifested bruises that became lesions and bled as an empathic response to recalling witnessing a neighbor being shot.[121]

Psychogenic purpura is similar to another bodily change through altering differentiation: a psycho-physiological mechanism identified in the medical profession that produces changes in the physical body, known as autoerythroctye sensitization. This medical condition occurs when patients become sensitive to their bleeding from a past trauma or accident, and reproduce that bleeding months and even years later in the form of spontaneous bleeding.[122] Blisters, a different bodily altering, have also been created during hypnosis, with suggestions of itching and extremely unpleasant emotional experience.[123] William Needles summarized a case of a blister created through hypnotically suggesting that a coin placed on the shoulder of a subject was red hot. Hypnotic suggestion has also been reported to have created a nosebleed in a person.[124] Through hypnosis, Dr. Montague Ullman, a New York psychiatrist and psychoanalyst, produced herpes simplex lesions (like a cold sore) and reproduced a blister as a burn mark with a small flat file through hypnotic recall of an explosion during battle.[125]

Dr. Jim Tucker and others who have examined qualitative research on reincarnation show another interesting physiological change—the ability of the mother or the child to replicate marks and scars where injuries, assaults, and intrusions on the body occurred in a past life.[126] Experiments occur where a person marks a dead relative's body, requesting that he or she reappear with a mark in the place where the markings were made in her next life.

Physicians examining the stigmatics addressed the issue of the potential for self-inflicted wounds in several cases. Dr. Pierre Janet, a French psychologist and neurologist, sealed a foot in a copper shoe with a glass window, and Dr. Warlomont used a glass cylinder to successfully demonstrate that the wound was not self-inflicted.[127] The medical and psychological communities often diagnose such hard-to-explain phenomena as psychophysical diseases or pathologies, such as hysterical conversion or schizophrenia. Richard Lord asserted that secondary gains or psychodynamic aspects of suffering of the stigmata included avoidance of sexuality, avoidance of being a girl, excessive menstruation, and a punishment for guilt of incest wishes.[128] The fact that these demonstrations that the mind and perhaps the spirit can alter the body remain ignored speaks volumes about our perceptual limitations.

The altered levels of awareness for stigmatics during trance, ecstasies, or raptures remain largely ignored and mysterious. Dr. F. A. Whitlock, professor of psychiatry at Royal Brisbane Hospital, Australia, and J. V. Hynes perceived altered consciousness as having a "facilitatory effect on the production of changes that culminate in bleeding from open wounds in the skin."[129]

There are others who see the stigmata as a supernatural manifestation of God in the world. One explanation included a process of raising the lowest members of society to the position of power of the wounded healer through physical and emotional suffering at the hands of other worldly beings. Richard Lord stated:

> given the proper mental state there is no organic reason why bleeding 'wounds' cannot appear spontaneously at specific site although the physiologic mechanism is not known.[130]

Dr. Oscar Ratnoff, medical doctor, concluded, "Where mind and body meet, we all must recognize our ignorance."[131]

OUR RESPONSIBILITY TO EXPAND AWARENESS

The use of the human mind as a tool of perceptual awareness is a spiritual gift we all possess. Our own development of inner resources rather than blind allegiance to external forces is the goal of most forms of spirituality. "But better hypnotist than messiah," stated American writer Richard Bach,[132] pointing out the power of meaningful self-understanding versus exterior control by others.

Expanding our perceptual awareness with hypnosis includes expanding our connections and boundaries beyond what we may have been taught when dealing with spiritual aspects of our lives. If hypnotic, paranormal, or psychic abilities and spiritual gifts have been given to people to help others, then I believe those heroic individuals should follow their paths and help others to expand their Universes. Jesus often spoke of his father's house having many mansions, which you could interpret as meaning many paths to spiritual destiny. The words of Jesus seem fitting here, "Whatsoever you do to the least of my brothers that you do unto me." I interpret that statement to mean that we must include every human being and living creature on the face of the earth in our awareness and interactions. What I believe is the highest spiritual principle was expressed by Jesus, "Love thy neighbor as thyself." If you truly knew how to love yourself, you could do nothing less than love your neighbor.

Expanding your Universe involves developing a broader relationship to the world at large. You need to have a commitment to all life on earth and in the Universe, as your very existence (and the existence of the species) depends on the balance of nature. In this way, you will increase your empathy for all of life.

Animals become a part of our expanded consciousness. There are children and adults who have reported an ability to communicate with animals. They report that animals show them how they were abused by other people, how their families were taken from them, and how their spirits return and stay with other living animals. Some individuals might like evidence of the validity of these statements, but attempting to validate them quantitatively would likely only lead to futile attempts at controlling these aspects of life.

Let me recount a personal experience that involved subtle communication with animals. I remember once walking through the woods with a lover. She and I came upon a pasture with many deer, including many fawns, bucks, and does. They grazed and looked at us, never leaving or giving any signs of feeling unsafe. We sat down to enjoy their company. When two men began to walk up the road, the deer silently disappeared, and these men never knew that twenty deer had been grazing in this pasture. Did these animals realize that while we were harmless, the two men might be more aggressive? Did these animals (and do others) perceive the feelings of humans? Dorothy Bradley and Robert Bradley, both medical doctors, stated: "There are innumerable records of animals howling, refusing to eat, and showing other reactions coincident with the death of their beloved masters, even though separated by great distances."[133] A friend of mine, Georgie, called upon dolphins in the ocean waters of Florida where they had not been observed, and soon after, a number of them appeared. There are also many amazing stories of pets and other animals saving peoples' lives. Can they communicate in more complex ways with each other and other living creatures than people are aware of? After an experience like the one described here, I would certainly say that there is evidence they do realize when people might be intent on harming them, and they do possess sometimes uncanny levels of awareness, as well as abilities to communicate.

Clearly some aspects of the Universe remain unexplored and untapped and, while perceived by some, are nonexistent to others. Whether or not people can perceive paranormal and spiritual abilities in themselves and others does not stop such events from occurring in human lives and in the Universe. A quote cited by Dr. Abraham Maslow is apropos here, "As George Lichtenberg said of a certain book, 'Such works are like mirrors; if an ape peeps in, no apostle will look out.'"[134] This statement could describe perceptual hypnosis, since it is the individual's innate ability to access and seek out knowledge of self and the Universe that allows the person to bring special abilities into conscious awareness and under conscious control, ultimately putting that person more spiritually in touch with self. These abilities are a birthright, but have been socially conditioned out of the conscious control and perceptual awareness of many individuals.

A hypnotist might use hymns and scripture in his methodology—drawing Christian or other religious imagery into hypnotic experience. Ethical hypnotists always shape hypnotic experience to a client's particular chosen perceptions and personal meanings, rather than to their own. So, if a client wants religious imagery, the professional can include it, but if a client is opposed to it, then the professional should leave it out. When it is appropriate for and acceptable to the client, a hypnotist could help to move religious images into higher levels of awareness in an individual's perceived Universe. During hypnosis, an individual might visualize or perceive Jesus or God as touching his or her life, cleansing his or her soul, and healing his or her troubles and everyday problems.

In 1984, Dr. William Nicholas Curtis founded the National Association of Clergy Hypnotherapists for professionals, an ecumenical and educational organization that expanded the applications of hypnotherapy. Dr. William Kroger, an American medical doctor who pioneered the use of hypnosis in medicine, pointed out that numerous well-known Catholic physicians and psychologists have contributed to the medical and mental health fields with hypnosis.[135] The same is true of other faiths.

Dr. Rachel Copelan, a medical hypnotist, indicates that in keeping with Christianity, many clergy are using hypnosis because "Biblical teaching tells us all healing power is derived from God."[136] William Joseph Bryan, an American hypnotist, compared hypnosis to enhancing Christian principles.[137]

Reverend Irving C. Beveridge, Pastor of the First Baptist Church in Marshfield, Massachusetts, wrote a book on the Christian aspects of hypnotherapy. He stated:

> The mindset of the Christian to receive the message of the Lord through the media of hypnosis, when formed, is so convincing an argument to do what I do, that I wonder why I never did it earlier, and why indeed I waited as long as I did before venturing down the fascinating and faith-lined paths of hypnotherapy, either self-hypnosis or guided therapeutic hypnosis. If, as I maintain, Jesus was the master hypnotherapist, then his methods should indeed be more than adequate for the Christian to pursue and engage in.[138]

In keeping with Reverend Beveridge's endorsement of hypnosis, experience has shown that prayer and meditation also alter your level of awareness. An altered level of awareness, often associated with hypnotic experience, is mentioned in

Biblical scripture. When experienced in both prayer and hypnosis, altered awareness is often referred to as "being in a trance," where all sense of time and space is changed. Acts 22:17 states: "And it came to pass, that, when I came to Jerusalem, even while I prayed in the temple, I was in trance."[139] Other passages also connect prayer and trance. C. Bernard Ruffin, author, pointed out how Padre Pio stated that praying for your ancestors transcended time and space, as the present and past were occurring simultaneously. Padre Pio emphasized that in the present you can pray for the happy death of your great-grandfather.[140]

For persons to restrict their perceived Universe to limited experience and rigid differentiations based on religion, the Bible, or a pre-existing philosophy would be like physically eating only one type of food and never daring to taste anything else. As Dr. Egan, professor of psychiatry and organizational studies at Loyola University of Chicago, stated: "Although causes empower people, we should beware when a person believes that all he or she needs to know is in one book,"[141] referring to those who restrict their knowledge and openness to life to whatever is said by one source, such as the Bible. Keeping an open mind about what hypnosis can do for you can bring a richness to your life, like bringing a buffet of tasty new food choices to the table.

In secular circles, too, an increasing number of psychologists are adding hypnosis to their clinical practice, and are conducting research on hypnosis, expanding its application in the field. These applications have removed significant suffering from many individuals' lives.

EVIL: A FEAR AND PERCEIVED THREAT

When a fanatic and zealot begin to demonize or label as evil those things that are unknown, feared, or simply in opposition to their own opinions, they create a dangerous situation. Although spiritual gifts and innate human potential are available to all as a birthright, in the case of zealots or fanatics, religious or spiritual faith reflects their suspicion of anything deviating from their currently perceived ideas and beliefs. Such individuals have a restricted and narrowed perceived self and Universe. The bigger picture is imperceptible to those who have removed so much from their perceptual awareness of the world.

An inexplicable phenomenon is often labeled as a delusion, mirage, apparition, or hallucination. The problem with such labels is that the person using them is indicating that he or she feels a threat to his or her existing perceived self and Universe. Such a perspective needs to be examined, expanded, and reorganized—to experience and encompass new aspects of perceptual awareness and bring them into higher levels of awareness. This expansion can be hard to achieve, unfortunately, because changing the self can be threatening and scary to the restricted person.

After you begin to expand your perceptual awareness, spiritual experiences may appear more real than even everyday experiences; for example, vibrant colors can appear more clearly and intensely than usual. A faith that restricts perceptual awareness manifests that the faith itself suffers from a degree of inadequacy, its ideas threatened by the unknown. As Matthew Fox, American priest theologian, stated during an interview with Sam Keen, a writer for *Psychology Today*, "If we were healed we would stop living in our tiny world of 'do's and don'ts' where we are saved and no one else is, and we would start living in a Universe that had a hundred billion galaxies."[142]

A perceived sense of superiority with a desire to have authority over others or to control others is just what Jesus warned against. And such behavior is more a reaction out of fear and ignorance than anything else. Unfortunately, such attitudes are expressed by authority figures in many occupations, and you need to understand their source and their true essence—how they are like the threats of mind control and brainwashing discussed earlier. Such views often remain unchanged and rigid, even when the person's perceived Universe reveals that these outdated points of view are a distortion of a greater truth. That person must make an attempt to understand and respect another's tradition, rather than being tempted to competitively outdo it in defense of what might seem like the superiority of his or her own ideas or life path. As an example, American author Joseph Chilton Pearce reported the following incident from the Hindu fire-walking ceremony honoring the god Kataragama in Ceylon:

> Of the eighty people walking that night, twelve failed. Some required lengthy hospitalization and one man was burned to death. The devout dismiss these accidents. Those people, Feinberg was told, simply lacked faith or proper preparation. Feinberg then related the fate of a young English missionary who was quite upset by the ceremony and vowed to walk the fire next time, to show Christian faith to be as firm as Hindu. He did walk the fire, somehow, and spent the next six months in the hospital where doctors barely managed to save his life.[143]

The narcissistic (self-centered) action of this English missionary was based on his distorted perceptions of another's spiritual path. A narcissistic point of view is based on an inadequate and narrow image of God projected to fit the person's needs and perceptions of life. It is both culturally and spiritual insensitive and leads to harm in many ways. Such was the case in the witchcraft trials in Salem, Massachusetts, in the 1600s, where a number of innocent people were put to death in the name of God. It seems even in today's society many people are trying to influence your free will to bolster their own beliefs or for their own benefit, often without your best interests in mind, and using hypnosis without your consent.

So-called righteous persons maintain perceived selves that are inconsistent with the definition of an adequate personality advanced by perceptual psychology and demonstrate a high degree of inadequacy by persecuting others. Dr. William James's presented a case of a magistrate in Bamberg, Germany, between 1627 and 1631, accused of being a warlock and making a pact with the devil. The magistrate defied his accusers and pointed out that these accusers who tortured him were the devils themselves. Dr. William James concluded that the so-called witches were victims and the accusers were perhaps the insane and possessed.[144]

Perceptual awareness explains that you perceive things through more than just your physical eyes. As Dr. Frederick Franck, a Dutch artist, stated: "He who sees, understands Christ's "I am the Light of the World" and the Buddha's "I am the Eye of the World." And he who knows it is all in the SEEING, understands from the Upanishads: Not what the eye sees, but that which makes the eye see, that is the Spirit; and "Truly, oneself is the Eye, the endless Eye."[145]

This quote reminded one colleague of the Grateful Dead song, "Eyes of the World," and the lyric, "Wake up to find out that you are the eyes of the world." These passages also support the notion that the potential for expanded perceiving is very spiritually based and involves changing perceptions and personal meanings from more than just a physical or mental perspective.

It is not advisable to go into complete darkness without a flashlight of some sort. You can think of hypnosis as providing that light. It is never too late to experience something new when you have such a potential existing within you. A better understanding of hypnosis can empower you to see life with its many spiritual aspects at higher levels of awareness in your perceived Universe, to be more open to new experiences, and to identify with others more fully.

A number of other approaches to understanding human experience have utilized hypnosis, such as Christian hypnotism, the Jungian approach to hypnosis, and existential hypnotherapy. Whatever the approach, all are derived from perceptual awareness, and are a consequence of a person's personal history and present need to maintain and maximize personal potential. Perceptual hypnosis is one way to help you and other people travel down that path.

PERCEPTUAL POINTS

- Clearly some spiritual aspects of the Universe remain unexplained and untapped and, while perceived by some, are nonexistent to others.
- Christians have provided quite a bit of evidence of the acceptance and effectiveness of hypnosis when combined with Christian symbolism and

beliefs. Jesus advocated for increased awareness in individuals rather than the blind following of others.

- The perceived self can be either expanded or restricted, depending on a person's perceptual capacity for differentiation.
- Hypnosis has created physical changes in the human body through altering a person's perceptual awareness. Stories of such physical changes demonstrate a capacity for control over the physical body by the mind and spirit that people are taught is not possible, despite the acknowledged existence of the stigmatics.

PERCEPTUAL EXERCISES

1. Self-examination: If your boss is perceived as controlling by you, look for where you are controlling in your life. If your spouse is _____, in what way are you also like that? Then think about how these behaviors began and what you can do to change them in yourself.

2. What are your spiritual strengths? And how are they also your weaknesses? List them and journal about the positives and negatives. Now ask someone close to you to describe your strengths and weaknesses. Compare and contrast your views and the other person's views. See if you can understand where they are coming from in their descriptions.

3. Religion and spirituality: List the common characteristics between your religion or spirituality and someone else's, then compare your perceptions of the positive and negative qualities of your views to those of someone with a different background whom you are close with.

4. Journal how you have changed your views as a result of these exercises.

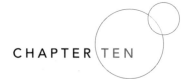

CHAPTER TEN

PARANORMAL AND OTHER SPIRITUAL PHENOMENA AND PERCEPTUAL HYPNOSIS

When we are well and healthy and adequately fulfilling the concept "human being," then experiences of transcendence should in principle be commonplace.[146]

—*Dr. Abraham H. Maslow*

Spiritual experiences lead to an evolved and deeper understanding of life and unexplained phenomena that challenge our everyday knowledge of how the Universe works. Hypnosis is one bridge to that knowledge. More people than ever are now reporting psychic, paranormal, and spiritual experiences. Everyone has psychic abilities, but only a few people are really tuned in to them. These "gifts" occur across a range of ages, all levels of education, all socio-economic classes, both sexes, and all races. Historically, the study of paranormal, psychic, or spiritual phenomena began in the United States with the establishment of the American Society for Psychical Research, in 1885, under the directorship of Dr. Richard Hodgson. This chapter presents paranormal experiences, such as recalling past lives and near-death experiences, along with cases of energy zappers known as "spiritual vampires" (because they suck the life out of others). It also examines themes of spirituality, including oneness and the many multicultural aspects of this theme, as well as how spirituality is phenomenologically defined and how it is related to your inherent connection to other visible and invisible aspects of the Universe and their blurred union.

An expanded view of the self and the Universe occurs through spiritual and paranormal experiences. Dr. William Roll, a former psychologist and member of the faculty of the Psychology Department of the University of West Georgia in the United States, and a noted parapsychologist since the 1950s, spoke of how awareness of paranormal experiences can help people redefine the boundaries of the self: "one way of looking at ESP (Extra Sensory Perception) and PK (Psychokinesis) is to regard them as evidence that the human self extends into the environment in ways that have not so far been brought out by science."[147] Dr. Roll went on to say: "Most systems of psychotherapy do not recognize that the human organism extends into the space beyond the skin, and, therefore, they lack techniques for bringing this part of the self into awareness."[148]

Paranormal aspects of our lives continue to interest people and stretch their rigid and outdated views of the Universe. For example, can someone astral-project into your private space at any point? Do ghosts or spirits view you in your most intimate moments? Some signs of ghosts that are commonly reported in my research include:

- A moving shadow
- A formless light
- Hearing your name called
- Hearing footsteps or knocking on doors or walls
- Doors opening by themselves
- The smell of food, tobacco, perfume, flowers, something burning, or a foul odor
- Feeling you are being watched or are not alone
- Lights bulbs flashing on and off
- Telephones ringing with strange synchronistic messages
- Doors being locked or unlocked in ways that remain unaccountable
- Items disappearing and then reappearing

Other questions arise, such as, are telekinetic powers responsible for some physical illnesses, accidents, and tragedies? The interesting truth is that if paranormal phenomena exist and affect the Universe, ignoring such occurrences does not change the fact that they exist and shape your experiences, whether you are aware of such influences or not.

Surveys conducted in the last thirty years show that it is more common than once thought for individuals from all walks of life to have had some kind of a psychic or spiritual experience.[149, 150] Such reports are signposts of how the perceived Universe is changing for many people. Perhaps in the future even more people will have these experiences, in keeping with Professor Robert A. Campbell's statement that: "The higher attainments of the exceptional few in any age, is only the prophecy of what will, in some succeeding age, be the general attainment of the fairly average human being."[151]

The principles of perceptual hypnosis suggest a developmental process or an expanding Universe for those who slowly discover and develop psychic and paranormal abilities that may have been lost through the current socialization process. In socialization, as a child, you psychologically and physically became aware of self as a separate being from that of your parents. By contrast, in a spiritual awakening you begin to realize your unity or oneness with the Universe. This awakening may at first induce terror and fear of intrusion by negative forces. Generally though, through divine sources and interventions, you develop a spiritual individuality simultaneously with a feeling of safety. A sense of hierarchy disappears because all differentiations within the Universe suddenly have equal importance. For example, in order for life to exist, all aspects become important. A plant needs the sun, the clouds, the earth, and your exhaled breath. As boundaries collapse you begin to realize the unity between the many aspects of the Universe. This unfortunately applies to the perilous state of our environment also. Toxic waste in one part of the world will inevitably affect other parts of the Earth.

Paranormal experiences seem to be the result of abilities that only some people have developed or mastered. These abilities may be expanded through a blurring of your external and internal boundaries or aspects of your perceived Universe in a way that allows for a wider perceptual field and a more accurate perceptual awareness of the Universe.

Paranormal experiences may include:

- Telekinesis—the influence of the mind on other living or nonliving things
- Telepathy—perceiving another person's feelings, thoughts, or life events without the physical senses
- Clairvoyance—seeing something at a distant place
- Contact with poltergeists, spirits, and ghosts
- Alien abductions
- Retrocognition—seeing past events in the present
- Precognition—seeing the future while awake and in dreams
- Trance channeling/mediumship—becoming a conduit for a spirit guide, deceased person, or other entity to communicate for them

It is important that individuals who experience such paranormal phenomena understand key aspects of such experiences. It is also important that they know that they are not alone, that others share common reactions to such experiences. For example, precognition can cause individuals to blame themselves, wondering if their dreams and visions of the future helped create the experiences. Their feelings of fear or guilt are often compounded when the person warns others who ignore the warning. Those who were warned often blame the messenger for the tragedies that occur. In some instances, thank goodness, a warning can help people avoid danger or prepare them for what lies ahead.

One paranormal experience that can produce panic or fear of death when it first occurs is a spontaneous out-of-body experience. During the first two times I left my body spontaneously after hypnotic training, I slammed back into it after looking down from a few yards above my body, hovering in the room. I felt that my presence was not in my body but in my perceptual awareness that was observing it. It was as if I was seeing as I see out of my eyes but not from my eyes. Dr. Elena Gabor, a Doctor of Stomatology in Europe and certified hypnotherapist, pointed out that according to near death research, our consciousness does not originate from our brain but from that which existed before our bodies.[152] My immediate thought was, "What's going on here?" Although I sought out this experience through self-hypnosis, I still felt some fear at that time.

When you experience this situation, what you need most is reassurance that you are not "going crazy." Understanding that others have had similar experiences helps you adjust to this expanded perceptual awareness. Unwarranted psychiatric or psychological interventions or medication may cause more harm than good, and only alienate healthy and adjusted individuals from psychology professionals. If a psychologist denies the reality that out-of-body experiences occur, that doesn't help his or her client sort out what is going on and, in effect, invalidates the client's experience.

An expert hypnotist experienced with such phenomena can help distinguish genuine paranormal experiences that are externally influenced from those that are internally self-created. As a consequence, peoples' reactions can become stabilized and their fears that they are "going crazy or being psychotic" can be removed. They will gain an understanding of these new aspects of their perceived Universe that changes their reality and reduces anxiety. By sharing the paranormal event with others who've had similar experiences, clients reduce their sense of social isolation. A hypnotist provides support and empathy to counteract the negative reactions of those who maintain more restricted possibilities and a more narrowed perceived Universe. As a result, persons who have had paranormal experiences can comfortably explore their experiences with the hypnotherapist, rather than expend unnecessary energy attempting to justify them to those who don't understand or feel threatened by them.

To help you see paranormal experiences as less threatening, let's take a look at some characteristics that most such events have in common:

- Quiet mind
- Spontaneity
- Open-mindedness
- Identification with others
- Unity or connectedness

Paranormal phenomena usually happen unexpectedly or occur spontaneously. You require certain capacities in order to develop such gifts, such as being open-minded, having patience and anticipatory desire, identifying with others, and regularly practicing perceptual exercises to expand your awareness. Usually, these experiences happen when your mind is at peace, not filled with day-to-day concerns or busy with words and thoughts. Your mind is just silent. It is a slow and steady process of trial and error to develop and discover your particular talents.

Some individuals see results in days or weeks, and others take months before they see any benefit. Just as most people beginning a fitness program cannot enter a gym and begin to lift the maximum weight on the first day, and just as a woman typically doesn't give birth until the proper development of the fetus inside her has occurred, a client developing paranormal potential has to start with small steps to get validation, create an atmosphere of success, and progress gradually toward greater goals.

Paranormal or psychic abilities have great implications for how you define your perceived self, your personal world, and the Universe. Kennedy, Kanthamani, and Palmer reported that people with artistic creativity and evidence of spiritual beliefs had increased incidences of psychic and spiritual experiences, while those who focused on accumulating wealth reported fewer incidences of psychic phenomena.[153]

Paranormal and psychic phenomena usually occur during a feeling of calmness and relaxation with a clear and quiet mind. Fear of anticipated negative judgments of others is sometimes a first reaction to the experiences. Paranormal abilities can produce fear as people realize that previously held false views of reality are being stripped away and a paradigm shift is occurring.

Many people believe that spiritual and paranormal abilities are normal and that the human race has just forgotten they possess them. Perhaps that is what Jesus was pointing out when he said that "the kingdom of God is within you." Many everyday experiences can validate your inner resources but remain forgotten, because they are outside of what you normally differentiate. Dr. Erickson stated that "the so-called paranormal powers and miraculous healing were simply activated states of normal psychophysiological processes."[154] Raymond Moody, MD, the near-death experience researcher, agreed with Erickson and stated during a conversation with me, "There is no parapsychology; these are normal abilities and functioning of the mind."

Many psychic phenomena are experienced while an individual nonlinearly perceives external aspects of his Universe. For example, Dr. Moody shared the following about near-death experiences:

> my informants agree that the review almost always described as a display of visual imagery, is incredibly vivid and real. In some cases, the images are reported to be in vibrant color, three-dimensional, and even moving. And even if they are flickering rapidly by, each image is perceived and recognized. Even the emotions and feelings associated with the images may be re-experienced as one is viewing them.[155]

In addition, Ian Stevenson, MD (1987) stated:

> Persons who nearly die and then recover report having had perceptions— some of them not greatly different from their ordinary ones—even though their physical bodies were ostensibly unconscious and sometimes thought to be actually dead, although they were not. Their sensory experiences, which seem to be had from a position in space different from that of their physical bodies, are not mediated by normal processes of the sensory organs.156

There are cases of people, with their physical eyes closed and hovering near death, reporting accurately exactly what occurred in an operating room, seeing it from above or from one side of the room. A variation on this nonlinear experience of time is also described by near-drowning individuals who say that their life "flashed before their eyes." This process of viewing one's life events has been called panoramic memory. Another hypnotic phenomenon that occurs nonlinearly is known as time distortion, experienced as long durations of life experiences occurring in the present or re-occurring from the past in a few seconds.

DEBUNKERS: IGNORING SUBJECTIVE EXPERIENCE

A need for change is noted through the application of the scientific method in particular areas of study. The scientific method is criticized by some professionals because of its inability to grasp nonlinear experience, such as hypnosis, altered levels of awareness, or even love. Rene Descartes, a French philosopher, discovered the scientific method as a result of a dream after meditating all day long to discover his mission in life. Dreams are images of internal perceptual awareness. Descartes's story is rather ironic since many modern advocates of the scientific method in research deny the existence of internal experience and explain human behavior as stemming from measurable environmental or biological factors, which they claim are the only truly valid or provable means of conducting scientific exploration.

Yet Descartes's discovery is not so unusual. Many scientific discoveries began as internal images. Images perceived during twilight moments between sleeping and awakening are called *hypnopompic* (in the process of waking up) and *hypnagogic* (in the process of falling asleep) images. Such internal experience can be reproduced during hypnosis when a person has practiced imagining regularly. One famous internal image of a snake grabbing its own tail during a dream led to the discovery of a benzene ring by Dr. Friedrich August Kekule in Germany.

Clinicians often do not validate or understand many internal experiences and, while diverse meanings are often available to individuals, they are restricted when those in positions of authority cannot expand their perceived Universes to differentiate new aspects of experience. This situation causes clients who believe in paranormal or psychic phenomena to become confused and to not want to share their experiences with professionals. Some persons' internal experiences merge with external events in the Universe. Some people have found that this merging has resulted in their experiencing psychic or paranormal events. For example, a woman hugs her friend and has a thought alien to her that her friend's husband is going to make an attempt on her friend's life. This research participant becomes angry with herself about having such a thought without any adequate reason for such a thought to happen within her. Later the husband kills his wife, and the research participant struggles when her internal and external perceptions becomes united in reality.[157]

Other professionals validated psychic phenomena and spiritual experiences in therapy.[158, 159, 160, 161, 162] Several authors have reported instances of telepathic communication between therapists and clients. I can give an example from my own experience. I was working with a transvestite and attempting to understand his complex dynamics and psychology on a particular day. Later that day, a twelve-year-old girl who I had developed an excellent rapport with, came into my office. She promptly sat down and stated: "You should not be thinking about a man wearing dresses!" There were no reading materials or anything else in my office that would have suggested such thoughts. Coincidence? Perhaps. Rather than brushing this girl's statement off as an event with no explanation, I would be more likely to call this a situation in which the twelve-year-old was intuitively aware of her therapist's internal experiences—something that happens more often than people realize. As Dr. James W. Woodard, a sociologist from Temple University, stated back in 1935:

> The hazard of error in privately held worlds of meaning furnishes the reason why science insists upon public conceptual systems and experimental method. However, the individual scientist, especially the user of the artistic methods, should not be over-cautious in such a matter. His private scientific system may be more cogent than that which has as yet been publicly demonstrated; and the fault may lie only in the inability as yet to render objective what is subjective.[163]

Such creativity in an individual helps bring change and healing to the world.

Dr. Jerome Frank stated: "In fact, it seems plausible that one mode of transmission of the therapist's influence may be telepathy."[164] Dr. Cook further stated: "It is possible to communicate our thoughts to others without words or gestures or physical means of any kind."[165] Carl Sextus demonstrated that he was able to influence his clients from a distance beyond their physical proximity or without using their traditional sensory system—hearing, seeing, touching, and tasting.[166] Although a person's thoughts may be actively communicated to others, and others may be receptive when their thoughts are communicated to them, the form of the message may be varied, since a person could transmit images, feelings, thoughts, and other aspects of perceptual awareness telepathically.

The Amazing Kreskin (George Joseph Kresge), a famous stage mentalist in the 1970s to 1980s, discovered an ability to find hidden objects as a child. I witnessed his show in my hometown with my grandfather William Abel. He was escorted off stage in his finale, but returned to find his check, which had been passed around in the crowd and hidden by someone in the audience.

Since then, Patrick Wanis, another hypnotist, pointed out that no one has claimed the $100,000 he has offered to anyone who can prove under controlled conditions the existence of a "hypnotic trance."[167] How could anyone prove a trance since, as Kreskin and I both assert, hypnotic experience and psychic phenomena are simply altered forms of a person's perceptual awareness of the Universe, changes in differentiation that occur inside the mind?

I also stumbled on a book by Drs. Marks and Kammann, who expressed the belief that Kreskin was a hoax. I fail to see how Kreskin could have pulled off any hoax when police officers escorted him backstage; I can only guess that he used a form of perceptual awareness to find the person hiding the check. It would seem quite paranoid to think the police department conspired to assist in a hoax. Whatever his ability, Kreskin was well-prepared, confident, and successful in what he did. Throughout their book *The Psychology of the Psychic,* published in 1980, Marks and Kammann reiterated how they could not replicate any parapsychological findings. (How could you replicate a Kreskin performance, since few people have honed those abilities?) It quickly becomes apparent that they began with the premise of debunking all of parapsychology and created this reality for themselves. They are quintessential skeptics who refuse to expand their perceived Universes. The recent release of numerous people from prison's death row after DNA testing found that the physical evidence used to convict them was inadequate makes me wonder about what other atrocities have occurred in cases where objective measures fall short or when subjective experience that might be revealing is ignored.

Perhaps there is a spiritual reason why some people are unable to access their natural psychic and paranormal abilities. In regards to paranormal experiences, Dr. William James gave a great guideline and warning in 1902:

> The first thing to bear in mind (especially if we ourselves belong to the clerico-academic-scientific type, the officially and conventionally "correct" type, "the deadly respectable" type, for which to ignore others is a besetting temptation) is that nothing can be more stupid than to bar out phenomena from our notice, merely because we are incapable of taking part in anything like them ourselves.[168]

SPIRITUAL VAMPIRES

Another phenomenon of spirituality that is a focus of hypnosis and self-hypnosis is termed *spiritual vampires*, which come in all shapes and forms. This is one of the reasons for the need to protect yourself when doing any spiritual work or self-development. These entities are not the vampires of science fiction, but are people who suck energy from your body, mind, heart, and soul in order to accumulate resources and power. They suck out energy using hypnotic-like techniques to beguile their victims. Spiritual vampires also attempt to keep you from your goals and dreams. They feed off or drain your energy and your effort. Spiritual vampires may extract your energy consciously or unconsciously from four major channels of perceptual awareness: physical, mental, emotional, and spiritual.

The most basic technique of spiritual vampires on a physical or materialistic level is to use conscious mental strategies to deplete resources and energy from their victims to gain power and control over them. For example, here are some actions that might be viewed as spiritual vampire behavior:

- In a family or foster home, supplying basic resources to a potential victim but never enough to let the victim achieve independence and freedom
- As a customer, supplying just enough resources to bait the potential victim, but never actually granting the contract
- In intimate and family relationships, influencing people by stating beliefs that create fear and restrict awareness as facts, and fostering low self-esteem with toxic and negative comments

Spiritual vampires usually have no training and produce nothing, but use their time to get money from others, including skilled workers who provide services. They ostensibly offer tradespeople an opportunity to do their work or "friends" and associates a chance to attain their goals, but always with a cost hidden behind their carefully crafted hypnotic offer of false assistance.

The most dangerous vampires consciously use emotional and spiritual channels to extract resources of various sorts from victims. At such a level, a psychic vampire elicits fear and emotional arousal to confuse and tap a victim's energy. Such vampires are experts at seeing others' fears and weaknesses and using them to alter a targeted person's perceived Universe. They have strong internal barriers but excessively violate others' external boundaries, without any concern for their welfare. Such vampires often portray themselves as victims, as persons unjustly treated, or feign concern for you while they calculate how to improve their own interests and benefits through you.

There are also indirect vampires who shower gifts on one or two significant others while accumulating them from everyone else in their lives. These types of vampires are people

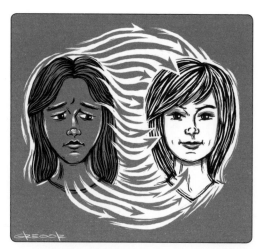

Spiritual vampire.

who take more than they give. Some spiritual vampires unconsciously drain others' energy, which may leave victims with feelings of being really tired after interacting with them.

Other vampires elicit rage and anger, while blocking healthy expressions of conflict resolution or problem-solving to further extract energy. They often restrict freedom of thought in others and sabotage positive external resources that would help their victims evolve or grow.

The regular practice of perceptual hypnosis and an understanding of how hypnosis works naturally defends you against spiritual vampire attacks on your being and energy. Learning the dynamics of perceptual hypnosis allows you to clearly see such manipulations and scams. Such differentiations allow you to protect yourself. Advertising today is often filled with lies about sales, effective products, and services from people acting as bloodsuckers rather than true service providers. These individuals and groups leave out relevant research that would reveal the illusions in their statements. Truth is stamped out, while falsehoods are validated, taking human beings farther and farther from their own natural birthright to truth.

Joe Slate, a licensed psychologist in Alabama, did some laboratory work that demonstrated changes in a person's aura, an energy field emanating from the body, due to psychic vampirism. He developed techniques to defend against such attacks and identified a number of types of psychic vampirism. He stated: "Anyone who lives by preying upon others can be seen as a psychic vampire."[169]

Conversely, genuine healers and clinicians often leave you feeling rejuvenated and refreshed. When genuine healers help others, energy is exchanged and flows naturally through the Universe. As a client, you walk away feeling relaxed and yet full of energy. Gauging how you feel after an encounter is one way to know if a practitioner is genuinely assisting you or just furthering his or her own needs.

OTHER PERCEIVED REALITIES

Life after death also becomes a focus in some paranormal experiences that involve perceptual hypnosis. Drs. Robert Bradley and Dorothy Bradley suggest an excellent approach to spiritual experiences and research, ". . . do a deliberate study via age regression under hypnosis of the subconscious awareness of those people brought back from clinical death! What a significant study this would be."[170] Dr. Michael Newton provided an excellent presentation of twenty-nine case studies of "life between lives,"[171] although he does not provide his age regression techniques from these partial sessions. He uses hypnosis to explore both spirituality and life after death. This new frontier gives humans glimpses of the memories of souls between reincarnations on earth.

Dr. Shakuntala Modi, an American psychiatrist, used hypnosis to uncover her patients' memories of creation.[172] Dr. Modi takes her clients back to the time of creation and helps them to understand or rediscover their spiritual evolution. She also focuses on possession experiences and used hypnosis to free individuals of external influences. Her results with hypnosis are usually the removal of her clients' symptoms. Uncovering memories can help you to expand your perceived Universe. You might see pursuing such studies as a stretch of the imagination, or might see them as a creative leap that can stimulate great minds of this century to push into unknown territory that has yet to be explored. To find your true spiritual path, you must begin by questioning everything, going down dead-end roads, rummaging through long forgotten pasts and unexplored emotions. Most important in any moment of time are attempts to understand the personal meanings that experiences have for you and attempting to develop perspective and perceive the Universe more accurately.

Another area of success with perceptual hypnosis is past-life regression. An interesting digression about past lives—the Christian Church endorsed reincarnation until the fifth century. The Gnostics, Clement of Alexandria and St. Jerome, spoke openly about it. Later in 553 AD, the Second Council of Constantinople ruled the doctrine of reincarnation as heresy. If you endorse a theosophical philosophy that explains that people have souls, reincarnate, experience karma and manifest souls through different bodies, you may act quite differently than if you think your actions end in the moment they occur. Although a controversial area of hypnosis, past-life regressions are quite popular.

In a past-life regression, you are regressed to another lifetime, grounded in the assumption that you have lived other lives before your present one. Some cases reported show interesting verifications. Unfortunately, past-life regression is difficult to validate and some believe it to be a result of suggestion, fantasy, imagination, wish fulfillment, and perceptions at lower levels of awareness in the present. Parapsychologists have explained some past-life reports as cryptomnesia, asserting that recall of information perceived in this life might actually come from various sources such as television, books, and other persons.[173]

Individual remarks about such experiences include:

- "You may think that I am deluded."
- "Actually, I'm not sure if those were past lives or just dreams no different from dreams you have at night."

The source of strange habits and fears may be traced to related experiences in other times. Fears, recurring illnesses, and strange habits attributed to past-life experiences include fear of blood, heights, going insane, thunder and lightning, and rodents. In some cases, applying knowledge of past-life circumstances gleaned from hypnosis has helped eliminate these habits and fears. Dick Sutphen, an internationally renowned hypnotist and author, demonstrated that engaging people with phobias and having them relive events from past lives in circumstances that caused these fears leads to the disappearance of the phobias.[174] Roger Woolger, PhD, a Jungian psychotherapist, uses past-life regressions to effect innovative psychotherapeutic change.[175] Dr. Edith Fiore, a clinical psychologist, and Dr. Brian Weiss, a medical doctor, have written extensively on past-life research. Using past-life regressions, hypnotists have also discovered patterns that seem to repeat themselves through a number of lifetimes, such as being abused in a past lifetime and again in this lifetime. These patterns echo some of the writing of Dr. Carl Jung, who spoke of a racial and genetic consciousness through which you gain memories of events that your ancestors lived through and a common knowledge of a time in history that may affect your present existence.

The continuing controversy between experts on this topic is amazing to observe. Recently, I reviewed an outstanding journal article about a validated case of past-life regression, in which a woman was able to recall minute and obscure details about historical facts that were popularly misrepresented, such as only two inquisitors being present in Cuenca, Spain, from 1584 to 1588 instead of three inquisitors. She corrected information on a building's location and provided the correct name of the Spanish governor. Linda Tarazi, a psychotherapist stated: "In spite of hundreds of hours of research on my part, no errors could be found." Linda Tarazi traveled to Spain and found the information (only two inquisitors) in the Episcopal archives, even after several professors had informed her that it had always been known there were three inquisitors at each tribunal. Linda Tarazi offers three possible explanations for the reports of this past-life regression in Spain:

1. Telepathy with a discarnate personality from 400 years ago
2. Possession by the one of the personalities in the past
3. Reincarnation[176]

What troubled me about this article was that Linda Tarazi cited the Bridey Murphy case,[177] in which a person relived a life in Ireland from the nineteenth century in the twentieth century. I had read other articles and books examining that case by Drs. Lawrence Kline and Melvin Gravitz, both professors at Georgetown University and prominent psychologists, and had already concluded that the Bridey Murphy case was a hoax.[178, 179] Believing what critical professionals on the Bridey Murphy case reported, I dismissed that case as untrue.

Drs. Kline and Gravitz's critical article had left me unaware, however, that psychiatrists Dr. Jule Eisenbud and Dr. Ian Stevenson had defended the evidence in the Bridey Murphy case. Later, after reading Linda Tarazi's summarization of the case, I discovered the Bridey Murphy case also had corroborated obscure verifiable information.[180] Struck by the confusion over whether the information was verified or totally unproven, I knew that I would have to read all the research on the case to determine the truth for myself, although it would require an extensive amount of time and study.

Drs. Kline and Gravitz also failed to mention the work of Dr. Curt J. Ducasse, a renowned professor of philosophy at Brown University. Dr. Ducasse revealed that the hypnotized subject had furnished a number of obscure details about Ireland, which had been verified and validated, including citings from a paperback published in 1808 that presented the meaning of the word "lough" and other information that Gravitz and Kline had dismissed prematurely.[181] Dr. Ducasse eloquently and intelligently demonstrated that critiques of the case by Christian theologians, newspaper and magazine reporters, and contemporary psychologists were unfounded. Those critiques unfairly debunked conclusions of the case that had been backed up by verifiable evidence. All of these debunkers felt threatened by the idea of reincarnation. Clearly, accurately perceiving events in our world is not so easy.

The battle to become aware of our Universe involves debates over differing viewpoints of what reality is and what is and is not in existence. Armed with perceptual dynamics and the qualities of the adequate personality, we will be in a better position to expand our boundaries.

PERCEPTUAL POINTS

- Paranormal experiences have been on the increase according to recent surveys. The principles of perceptual hypnosis suggest a developmental process or an expanding Universe for those who slowly discover and develop psychic and paranormal abilities that may have been lost through the current socialization process. The phenomenology of paranormal experiences is examined. Subjective evidence from debunkers is looked at from a perceptual approach and found to be identifying details that went unexamined.

- Together, the regular practice of perceptual hypnosis and acquiring a clear understanding of how hypnosis works naturally defend against attacks on your being that are coming at you on all levels of awareness through spiritual vampires.

- Various spiritual realities lead to an expanding of perceptual awareness and identifying with others in new ways.

CHAPTER ELEVEN

SUMMARY OF HYPNOTIC GUIDELINES AND AN EXERCISE TO HELP YOU APPLY THEM

Scientific progress showed that individual research and the freedom for individual scientific convictions do not prevent a large measure of scientific agreement.[182]

—Paul Tillich

Individuals of all sorts, from all different backgrounds, attempt to identify their problems and overcome them. By understanding the principles of perceptual hypnosis, people can increase the effectiveness of self-help tools, enhancing their physical, emotional, psychological, and spiritual well-being.

PERCEPTUAL HYPNOTIC PRINCIPLES

When individuals attempt to define their personal problems and solve them by applying perceptual hypnotic principles, their efforts require exploring their personal worlds and diverse Universe. That exploration further demands that the person identify essential aspects of their experience so as to perceive or differentiate diverse aspects of the Universe that they may have not noticed, including spiritual connections.

Drs. Donald Snygg and Arthur Combs define both diagnosing difficulties and searching for solutions from a phenomenological point of view as ". . . the exploration of the nature of the phenomenal field and of the differentiations that are characteristic of the field."[183] In other words, they look at the various aspects of meaning in a person's life. You and other people are all scientists, experimenting to find the most effective way to enhance your lives. You are all creating your own realities and must own responsibility for your lives so you can change what you don't like and bring more of what you desire into your lives. You may gain an expansion of your perceptual awareness as you begin to see the many perceptual possibilities in words and their meanings. Hypnotic experience, however, offers a concentrated and intensive manner of enhancing perceptual awareness and human experience in general.

As an individual, you search to find ways that enhance and improve everyday life. All self-help techniques can be explored from a viewpoint of your personal meanings and perceptions. You can turn the five principles for success with perceptual hypnosis discussed in the following sections into creative techniques, offering both everyday application and a search for opportunities to enhance your spiritual awareness and your individuality.

PRINCIPLE 1

By engaging in perceptual hypnosis, you can alter your perceptual awareness, expand your personal world, and increase perceptions available to you.

As you practice hypnosis, you increase the number and span of differentiations available to you. When you change your perceived Universe, you change your behaviors. For example, I once meditated on attracting money. The next day there were over 500 pennies on the front porch of my apartment. I have never had money on my porch before or since that moment when I mediated about receiving money. Somehow the combination of my inner thoughts and my outer world merged together, creating this event. Such incidents change how we see our world, the particulars of which must be worked out by each person individually on his or her path. You actually reorganize your perceived Universe by changing your differentiation of particulars in your environment, see newly perceiving aspects in your personal world, and bring aspects of the Universe that you were previously unaware of or not focused on into sight.

You seek to sustain or enlarge your personal world. Your personal world includes the not-self part of the field. But, of course, your perceived self is also an essential component. In your newly perceived Universe, instead of differentiating your limitations, you might, for example, focus on personal strengths and assets that help you live your life more adequately. Your freedom to examine any and all aspects of your personal world enhances your self adequacy.

PRINCIPLE 2

By changing how you see yourself in the Universe, you improve your ability to maintain and maximize your spiritual potential.

Changing how you see yourself improves your ability to maintain and maximize your potential. As Drs. Snygg and Combs pointed out, when you see yourself as inadequate, you misperceive aspects of your world.[184] Perceptual hypnotic experience might restore your damaged perceived self to a level of increased potential so that you can then perceive more effectively and behave accordingly. When you suddenly realize that you have the power to change your life, you then seem to participate in the world in a new way. You can re-incorporate aspects of your perceived self that you had perceived as not-self. Likewise you can remove unhealthy aspects that you had perceived as self that are not enhancing yourself, from your self-definition.

For example, one of my clients, a young girl, was told by a relative that she had bipolar disorder, a condition believed by some to be genetic. When this individual worked through inner changes with self-hypnosis and managed her emotions, it made it clear to her that she did not have bipolar disorder as she changed the perception of her body from damaged to healthy.[185]

While practicing perceptual hypnotic experience, you create new differentiations more consistent with a positive sense of self. Through hypnosis you can speed up growth, reducing the amount of time needed to perceive new aspects of the Universe. The process might create opportunities for you to open up to specific perceptions that you have avoided in prior weeks and months, possibly even years.

Milton Erickson's paradoxical strategies initially narrowed his clients' perceived Universes in an effort to create expansions of them. The process of telling stories allows individual images of your perceived self and Universe to come alive. While you are telling your stories, you creatively develop new perceptual potentialities that allow a more adequate perceived self to emerge into higher levels of awareness. As you change, so do many aspects of your everyday life. You might change your friends, job, and neighborhood. Sometimes you stay in the same place and make many new discoveries about your friends, job, or neighborhood that were once hidden from your view.

New experiences further change your self-definition and help create a new organization of your perceived self. For example, a person suffering from attention deficit disorder is asked during perceptual hypnosis to concentrate only on his hand. His response is that he can perceive his hand and all the feelings in his hand, including how his hand is touching the texture of his clothes. He is not able to concentrate on just his hand, but must bring his clothing into differentiation. This person had a history of overextending his perceptual awareness to include so many aspects of his Universe that he had difficulty concentrating on just one. Narrowing (squeezing out) these extraneous aspects of his perceived Universe was something he could not achieve in his everyday life without practice.

Perceptual hypnosis involves helping you to see your situation differently. The need to maintain and maximize your spiritual potential can only be addressed optimally when you are able to make ample and adequate differentiations in the Universe. As Erickson proposed, a positive experience occurring during hypnosis can have as great an impact on your perceived self as a past traumatic experience. When you face your fears and your false illusions, they vanish when you embrace a totally new perspective.

PRINCIPLE 3

Hypnotic experience gives you access to aspects of the Universe that were previously invisible.

Hypnotic experience makes accessible to you aspects of the Universe that have until now remained at low levels of awareness. Hypnosis provides a safe place to explore aspects of your perceived Universe. Through perceptual dynamics, hypnotic experience can allow you to accurately perceive more of your past. Normally, aspects of your Universe in higher awareness squeeze out less desirable perceptions, so that they go unattended. In a hypnotic state, you don't block out past experiences the way you do in everyday life. During hypnosis, you are not able to so conveniently forget or overlook an incident.

For instance, an eleven-year-old girl who had been raped was able to block out the entire experience for eight years. She had kept the experience at a low level of awareness all that time, but as she went through her teens, she found herself being fearful of men, especially men she found attractive. All of her relationships were negatively affected. When she went into hypnosis at nineteen, this client could bring the incident into a higher level of awareness and remember what had happened.

Hypnotic experience alters your awareness of aspects of your perceived Universe that normally remain hidden or unchanged. It allows a shift in your level of awareness. Those aspects of your perceived Universe that normally remain at low levels of awareness rise into higher levels of awareness during hypnosis, and you can then perceive them, just as my client who was raped finally perceived what had happened to her. A perceptually oriented hypnotherapist is then able to assist you in understanding your perceptual field dynamics. Drs. Snygg and Combs pointed out that although you remain unaware of their impact on your life, your perceptions at a low level of awareness affect future perceptions.[186] With assistance, you may be able to differentiate aspects of your perceived Universe that have long remained at lower levels of awareness, removing distorted or restricted differentiations and enhancing adequate ones.

PRINCIPLE 4

Perceptual hypnosis reduces unfounded threats to your perceived self so that you can differentiate and expand new aspects of your perceived Universe, unhampered by fear.

It is possible to have a hypnotic experience during which you accept threatening differentiations and your perceived self reorganizes. In addition, pseudo orientation in time can occur and possibly enable you to further reorganize your perceived

Universe to a moment before a trauma or problem entered your life or to a point in the future when this situation is resolved. Looking back on what once appeared threatening can be a different experience from dealing with it when it first occurred; you might see it as challenging or as totally harmless. For example, you may become fearful when you begin to realize that others may be able to perceive you when you are alone or be able to develop a telepathic link to your inner experiences. At first you may feel naked in a very vulnerable way until you realize a natural protection is available. Negative experiences may uncover your weaknesses and fears so that you can overcome them. Gradually you change your boundaries and relationship to the Universe, and likewise the Universe responds.

When self-esteem improves, situations or people who you have perceived as threats to self might no longer bring out that kind of response. Once you no longer feel the anxiety or fear of these situations or people, the need to defend a perceived inadequate self diminishes; instead, you can apply your energy to enhancing potential within yourself. Many ideas and concepts that were fuzzy and unclear can be brought into higher levels of awareness, and you can begin to clean up the clutter that holds you down.

In hypnosis, you can bring to the forefront experiences and perceptions you have been avoiding, go through the process of feeling that they are threatening aspects of your perceived Universe, and resolve these and related issues in a safe environment. Afterwards, the impact of such aspects is removed or reduced. In this way, hypnotic experience allows you to narrow or squeeze out negative aspects of your perceived Universe and expand your field of life by bringing more positive aspects of experience into higher levels of awareness.

 ## PRINCIPLE 5

Perceptual hypnosis allows multiple aspects of your perceived self to either emerge or be moved to lower levels, expanding or contracting your self-definition.

Perceptual hypnosis can lead you to accept the complexity of your perceived self, allowing various aspects either to emerge into higher levels of awareness or to submerge into lower levels. You can have an intuitive flash of insight that saves many lives one day and then lock yourself out of your house or car the next day. Even in the course of an ordinary day, your self-definition can expand or contract at any moment in time. Similarly, self-definition can change from social group to social group—as occurs when you act differently with different people and in different situations, acknowledging your multiple and contradictory natures as a spiritual being.

You then begin to communicate between these parts to create more harmony, acceptance, and balance within your perceived self. In so doing, you create a personality that is more diverse and flexible.

PERCEPTUAL PLAN: EXERCISES TO EXPAND PERCEPTUAL AWARENESS

In this chapter, I offer you an exercise to expand your perceptual awareness. In order to apply the many ideas and processes in this book, it's important to have not just intellectual awareness alone, but personal experiences as well. Therefore, do not drive or operate machinery when you conduct this exercise. Practicing daily to awaken your undeveloped abilities and make connections with your greater mind will be required. Slowly you will get in touch with your deeper knowledge and awareness. You can creatively imagine what you wish to experience and imagine that it will occur either spontaneously or through your creatively imagined practice. You enter such an experience by consciously quieting your mind or erasing your thoughts. Start by perceiving your physical body and all your inner feelings and experiences in this moment. Your feelings and images are aspects of your experience that need to be nurtured and repeatedly practiced. So, let us begin.

First, find a quiet place that you can go to once or twice a day to do this exercise. Next, find a relaxing position: it may be lying down on your bed or sitting in a comfortable chair or being in any other position on any piece of comfortable furniture that you would like. Make sure that you will not be disturbed by your cell phone or other disruptive noises from your environment. A great start is to focus so intensely that outside noises disappear. The more you can focus and block out the rest of the world, the more effective hypnosis will be. Alternatively, you can focus on a single external noise and, with practice, use it to bring you deeper into hypnosis. Over time, this is a necessary ability. If you have never experienced hypnosis, you may relax so much that you fall asleep, literally. You may experience itches and twitches of muscles, and may scratch your itch or just let it fade away. If you stick with this practice daily, in time it will give you much more energy, mental clarity, and calmness, even when you are faced with stressful situations. Clear your mind of any thoughts, or just notice the thoughts and let them pass through your mind as the wind passes through your hair or through the leaves on a tree. (There are numerous deep relaxation exercises you may use, all equally effective. They vary only in their verbal description and images, but follow the same outline and steps.)

Focus on a deep bright purple, with fluorescent sparks of violet. Imagine this color or another color you prefer with this same mixture of one shade deep and bright and another shade fluorescent, giving an effect of lightning bugs at night or glow-in-the-dark sparkling lights. First, take a deep breath. Count one, two, three, four, and five. Find whatever number is comfortable for you to breathe all the way in, deeply, fully, completely, and comfortably. Next, hold your breath to a count of three (or whatever that number is for you). Then, gently and slowly exhale completely to that acceptable number. Over time you may expand this to a count of four or five while holding your breath before breathing out and again before breathing in for this same count. Do this breathing exercise a few times and relax as much as possible. Breathe fully so that you let all the air in your lungs in and out each time you inhale and exhale. Let your breathing become natural. Imagine a third eye, a spiritual eye at the center of your forehead an inch above your eyebrows. Imagine that you can see in all directions, 360 degrees. If you cannot imagine this 360-degree view, imagine seeing as far around you as possible or fantasize that you are seeing this 360-degree view. You will notice that outside noises and your environment begin to fade away as you focus intensely on your internal world. Any outside noises simply bring you deeper, and you become more deeply relaxed. You can open your eyes in an instant and handle any necessary emergency effectively. Remember, you can just imagine in your mind's eye—you don't need to see with your eyes. For example, focus on an object or image for a few minutes. (Pause). Now ask yourself, "Was I aware of my hand?" No, you were not focusing on your hand, so your hand did not exist in your highest level of awareness at that time.

Close your eyes and let your eyes roll up in your head, looking at this third eye in the center of your forehead. This third spiritual eye can see from all sides: front, back, top, and bottom. Your third spiritual eye is like a library and storehouse. Everything you have ever experienced is recorded accurately and completely there and is available for you to see again, now, or at any time you desire. Your third eye connects you to your larger mind, your higher self, and its job is to be a recorder of your past, a protector and creator of your present, and a perceiver and inventor of your future. Your third eye helps you see things in new and different ways during hypnosis. At some point during your hypnosis, perhaps right now, perhaps in a bit, you will be looking out of this wondrous third eye as you continue to relax and go deeper. Now remember, your third eye records everything, guides you in every experience, and is an observer of, recorder of, and commander in carrying out all these suggestions. As it does its job, you will begin to notice something different in every experience you have while so deeply relaxed. You may feel your body getting heavier and heavier, like a heavy weight, or lighter and lighter, like a feather [choose your own images] floating through the wind. Perhaps your body begins to tingle or becomes numb. Your third eye perceives this suggestion, records, and carries out this suggestion.

Imagine as you close your eyes that these bright and fluorescent colors are moving slowly through your body as a fluid or as energy moving from your toes to the top of your head, swirling and massaging your being from the surface of your skin deep into your muscles and your bones and deeper into your inner self. Go slowly and allow each area of your body to relax and say in your mind, as you imagine this color purple moving up from the soles of your feet to your toes, "My soles and toes are so relaxed." See this energy soaking through and penetrating deeply into your body and being as a light illuminates a room or as a sponge absorbs water. A dry sponge is stiff and inflexible, but once filled with water, it expands and becomes soft and flexible. Imagine any tension in your muscles released. Imagine any negative energy as black specks and gray smoke that travels up through your body and exits through an opening on top of your head, rising into a ball. Notice your body and pay special attention to this mansion of your soul. It's odd how some people neglect to listen to their bodies. And you are listening to your body now. Notice your breathing, notice your heart beat, notice the different sensations and experience your body fully. Feel yourself relaxing more and more as the light you imagine moves up to the top of your feet and your ankles. Let the fluorescent sparks of violet light go wherever you feel tension, pain, irritation, or problems, allowing soothing, relaxing protection and healing into those areas. For example, if you have a broken bone or have a bruise or sore muscle, imagine these fluorescent sparks attracted to the spot that needs healing, just as moths are attracted to a street light. The fluorescent sparkles are soothing and enhancing your natural body's ability to heal those body parts. Imagine this for a few moments. Then imagine this colorful energy moving up to your lower legs, knees, and thighs.

See this energy moving through your genitals, your buttocks, your abdomen, your stomach, and your lower back. Feel how relaxing and soothing this colorful energy is to your treasured body. You are the protector and keeper of your body. You bring only nourishment and health to your body. Then move this energy up your fingers, palms and back of your hands, your wrists, your lower arms, your elbows, your upper arms, and up to your back and through your shoulders, merging to your neck. Go up through your stomach, chest, and back, and to your neck. Let your whole upper body relax. Imagine the muscles in your upper body relaxed. The energy moves deeper, into your bones. Your organs are relaxed and soothed and cleansed with this energy. You breathe in a healing energy, a natural medicine that mends and rejuvenates your airways and lungs. This energy spreads through your whole upper body, relaxing and calming you. Now your heart pumps perfectly, not too fast and not too slow—just right. Your emotions relax. Imagine all your neck muscles relaxing. Your jaw, face, and scalp and all the tiny muscles in your jaw, face, and scalp relax. Your eyelids become heavy. Your tongue relaxes. Your chin settles. Your scalp loosens. As this colorful light is moving up each part of your body, see any tension and stress as gray smoke or black specks or blobs leaving through the top of your head and forming a ball over your head. As you finish this relaxation, send this ball up into the sky and watch as it travels higher and higher. Just before it is out of sight, it disintegrates and vanishes into nothingness where it can no longer do you or anyone else any harm. Say to yourself, "And harm to no one."

Then see a ball of white light coming from the heavens and hovering over your head. Allow that ball of light to glow and grow. See it descend upon you and completely envelop your whole body just like an egg. See a spark of white light deep within you expanding and merging with this ball of light above your head. Feel this light enter your body and this ball of light merge with you, and allow yourself to think of nothing else but this ball of light, feeling completely peaceful, tranquil, and calm. You are completely protected and relaxed.

Imagine that you are walking on a beach. You feel the dry warm granules of sand between your toes. You see the blue sky. You feel the soft gentle breeze on your face and skin. You hear the ocean waves rhythmically come onto the beach. You smell the ocean air and feel a deep sense of relaxation entering your body, mind, and spirit. You see the sea gulls gliding through the air and hear their noises as they are moving about. You see the sunlight glittering off the ocean water. You walk down to where the water meets the land.

You imagine a gentle little wave splash up on your feet and ankles, bringing a warm wave of relaxation throughout your entire body. It feels so good to relax and let go. As each wave comes in, you feel this wave of relaxation. As each wave goes out, you feel the chains that block any obstacles to your self growth fall away and are carried out to the ocean, deep in the water where they are disintegrated and can no longer harm you. You can do this for as long as you like. Your true potentials are released as your restrictions and limitations are removed.

Imagine three scenes that are very relaxing for you, and be sure that during these scenes you felt very safe and secure with yourself in all ways or perhaps proud of yourself for something you accomplished. Take the first creatively imagined image, perhaps in some soothing water of a pool, or lake (if you are comfortable with water), or wherever you would like this place to be, and make an image of this place very vividly in your mind. Imagine everything about that scene: what it felt like, what you saw with your eyes, what you heard, perhaps what you smelled and tasted, and experience that scene from your past in your present, as fully and completely as you can. See this scene as vividly and clearly as you are able to. (If you do not visualize well, just think and feel it in your mind, even without the images, like day dreaming. If you are uncomfortable with water, pick another naturally soothing setting.) Take one particular image from this scene and label this "image 3." Next, take another scene from another time where you were very relaxed and pleased with yourself, say after you had completed a long and difficult project. As you are now enjoying a relaxing feeling after having finished your completed project, feel a sense of accomplishment and satisfaction of finishing a task, completing a goal, succeeding at what you set out to do. Take an image from this scene and label this "image 2." Take a more provocative and emotional scene of yourself as happily relaxed with a very positive self-image in your future, doing exactly what you have always dreamed of doing. See yourself in all aspects as happy and cherish this moment. Select an image from this scene and label this "image 1." Don't be concerned about how you will achieve this goal. When you are done with this image, just let it go like a ripple of water on a pond vibrating outward, until it disappears and is forgotten but forever exists in that moment and can be recalled when necessary. Each time you complete this relaxation with its colorful and fluorescent sparks, follow it with these three images, saying to yourself with each image, "I relax more and more."

Imagine the following colors as huge raindrops or protective bubbles that drop down on you or a shower of colored water that fills and surrounds you and bring you even more relaxing and tranquil feelings. Start with a red raindrop or protective bubble, and feel it penetrate every cell of your being while relaxing and calming you and making you more aware of your inner world. Then imagine an orange, a yellow, a green, a blue, an indigo, and a violet raindrop, or bubble or shower of water fill you. See, feel, and sense these colors vibrating brightly within and around you.

Now let's create your special place to work on your spiritual growth. See yourself traveling to this place. It can be an indoor place or an outdoor place. Create a comfortable spot to rest and a place where you can view images. Imagine in your place a mental collage of four pictures on a whiteboard, movie screen, written in some clouds, or on a ceiling if you are lying down in a room. (You might place a picture you have that reflects your ideal weight or appearance in your mirror or on a wall in your room, somewhere that you would see it every day.) For each picture you create, imagine that the more you look at it, the bigger, clearer, brighter, and more detailed it becomes, until it finally becomes a movie playing out in all its details.

Let your first picture be of yourself, as you want to be, maybe with a healed bruise or a little more or less weight. See brightness in your eyes, a glow on your face, and a gleam through your body. See yourself just as you wish to be.

In your second picture, create an image of a goal: for example, going to college, having a wedding, getting a job, going on a vacation, or completing whatever achievement you wish to accomplish. See yourself engaged in this activity. Notice all the details of your movements, how graceful and perfect they are.

In your third picture, place an object you wish to have or need: a specific book, a fact you wish to know and have been unable to find, a ring, increased income, a dress, or something like that. See the object, its color, and its texture— how it feels, perhaps its smell. See it in all its detail.

In your fourth picture for this mental collage, place an image of a relationship or person who is important to you. This relationship may be with someone you wish to improve your experience with, such as a boss, a family member, or a partner. See that person's face in a kind and happy image and, as this movie unfolds, see yourself as expressing authentic feelings of love, caring, and having a better understanding with the person you choose. Send him or her forgiveness or ask for forgiveness without words. Send these feelings and images honestly and openly in your mind, without using any words.

Next, allow your perceptions to be experienced and flow without a need to identify or hold on to them. Observe them like the wind blowing through your hair, or a summer's breeze blowing through leaves of a tree. Look for what you did not see in these experiences in your past. What are these feelings, thoughts, the bodily awareness, images, energy, and behaviors from these inner images? And how are you responding at this moment in time?

Say to yourself: "That part of myself that knows what's going on in my body, my mind, and our Universe, and which I don't allow myself to perceive or know, can communicate to me when I say I am as deeply relaxed as I have ever been, and even more deeply relaxed." That inner protector/creator is always aware. Find a secret word that you would never read in a book or hear someone say in everyday life and say that word to yourself now, "----." Say: "I feel myself rising higher and higher from my body into all of my perceptual awareness, where all my hidden and potential abilities manifest. My body and mind are open to all my perceptual awareness as I use more and more of my mind's potential each day. My everyday 'consciousness' merges with higher and lower levels of awareness." (As you say this, imagine two colors merging to make a new color, such as red and blue becoming purple.) "Dimensions of my mind watch, record, and create all these experiences in a way that is best for me and at a time that is best for me. My larger mind draws me like a magnet to experiences that help me achieve my goals. My higher self protects me and watches over me."

Quiet your mind, allow your thoughts to drift by you, and focus on your body. Make your mind a blank. Say: "I remove all barriers and there is no distance or clock time now." Remember the higher and lower levels of your mind's awareness are not just a closet of skeletons from your past, but a gold mine of possibilities and potential, awaiting your activation now and in your future. Say: "I open my mind, my spirit, and my body to its full potential now." Say: "I choose to activate my potential now." As you practice these exercises, you will develop a better ability to relax and tune into yourself and your perceived Universe.

Imagine that you can travel anywhere in your world and see yourself there. Imagine a very familiar room or place that you often visit. Concentrate only on that place and notice all of your senses opening to this place. See, hear, feel, and sense all that is there. Notice a color and what it looks like, how it makes you feel, what it sounds like and what it tastes like . . . Notice a piece of fruit (or something else if you don't like fruit) and perceive just what it tastes like to you . . . Smell a pretty flower perhaps a rose . . . Take a few moments and just explore this place and all that you experience here. Your hypnotic experiences will be enhanced and your potential stimulated. Say to yourself: "Each day I see something new in my life. I learn a new way of seeing things." Count in reverse of how you counted in the beginning, and as you reach the last number, open your eyes, awaken now, to your true potential. Write down your experiences and keep a written record of them.

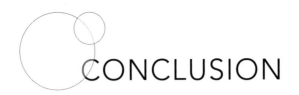

CONCLUSION

- Overall, hypnotic experience is created through altering your everyday perceptual awareness and expanding your perceived Universe. You choose to see and to experience, and you also choose not to see and not to experience certain aspects of your environment, your world, and the Universe.
- Many individuals suffer from *neopercipihypnophobia*, a fear of perceiving new experiences or of being de-hypnotized. I coined this word to express this fear of and inability to allow the self to create new perceptions and expand the ability to produce new thoughts, emotions, or behaviors that are unfamiliar. The fear leaves persons hampered by a restricted and narrowed view of the Universe.
- Perceptual hypnosis is a way to sharpen your awareness, to enhance your ability to accurately differentiate what is happening around you, and to improve your ability to determine what is influencing you. Perceptual hypnosis may assist you in completing those tasks that remain incomplete but are still active in your internal experience, thus freeing you to more fully experience your personal world while perceiving the Universe as accurately as possible.
- Perceptual hypnosis is an innate ability that you can use to expand your knowledge of yourself and the Universe, while preventing you from becoming easily influenced by external sources without your full awareness. Through a proper use of hypnosis, you can expand your perceptual awareness at higher levels and expand your knowledge of the Universe.
- All people must face their fears in order to evolve. An average person, uneducated and inexperienced in perceptual hypnosis, often believes just the opposite of what is conveyed here about hypnosis. How did these mistaken viewpoints arise? Such misinformation can come from those who already know how to easily influence you without your knowledge, or from those who fear change or demand the status quo remain the same or that others agree with their particular personal perception of the Universe. Yet too much agreement removes the very possibilities that would free your perceptual potential. You can remain perceptually unaware of any aspect of your perceived Universe in order to validate a prejudice or fulfill a wish.

I recommend that you experience hypnosis with a competent therapist who shares common aspects of your perceived world to determine the truth about hypnosis for yourself. After all, truth—accurate perception—will set you free. You must stand up to tyrants of any sort, move toward truth and freedom of expression, and seek the help of those heroic individuals who embrace your uniqueness and individuality.

One day while sitting on the beach with a friend named Bonnie, I began to feed some sea gulls. The sea gulls began to gather around us and completely encircle us. I noticed that my feeding basically elicited two types of responses from these sea gulls. Some sea gulls were much too afraid to come close to us. After making several false starts toward us, they would begin to squawk and make all kinds of noises. Other sea gulls would stare at us and quietly approach until reaching the pieces of bread on the ground close to us, and retreat after picking up the bread with their beaks. I invite the reader to follow the example of the latter sea gulls—instead of talking about negative aspects of hypnosis or the problems in your life, for that matter, do something. Experience hypnosis and obtain what you need to perceive accurately and to make your potential a reality in your life.

A pessimist sees the limitations in life, while an optimist sees potential waiting to be realized. Perceptual hypnosis demonstrates that we have much more potential lying dormant within us than many of us even realize. The inner depths of our being are still a new frontier to be explored. Get this picture. You perceive it and you can achieve it! Join those who realize that great powers and potential lie dormant within yourself and await your rediscovery.

PERCEPTUAL POINTS

- Perceive it and you can achieve it. Practice the perceptual hypnosis exercise provided in this chapter daily to work on expanding your perceptual awareness.
- Don't project—connect! Changing how you see yourself improves your abilities to relate to the Universe and maintain and maximize your potential and connections.
- Pioneer new territory! Hypnotic experience makes accessible aspects of your perceived Universe that have remained at low levels of awareness.
- The end is always a new beginning.

APPENDIX A: STIGMATICS

Over 321 stigmatics have been identified. These include:

Blessed Alexandrina Maria da Costa of Balasar, Portugal (1904–55)
Angela of Foligno
Anna Maria Taigi (1769–1837)
Anna Rosa Gattorno
Anne Catherine Emmerich, West Germany (1774–1824)

Camilla Battista Varani
Catherine de'Ricci (1522–89)
Catherine of Genoa,
Catherine of Racconigi, Dominican (1486–1547)
St. Catherine of Siena of Italy (1347–80)
Charles of Sezze
Christina Ciccarelli
Clara Isabella Fornari
Clare of Montefalco
St. Colette (1380–1447)
Cloretta Robinson (1962–)

Dorothy Kerin of London, England (1889–1963)

Elizabeth Achler Elena Ajello (1910–)
Elizabeth Canori Mora (1774–1825)
Elsie Nilsson Gjessing, married (1904–)
Enza Milano of Termini Imerese, Sicily, Italy (1938–)

Fausine Kowalska
Flora of Beaulieu
Frances of Rome
Saint Francis of Assisi, Italy (1186–1226),

St. Gemma Galgani (1878–1903)
St. Gertrude the Great, Germany (1263–1302)
Georgette Faniel of Montreal

Helen of Hungary

Jim Bruse

St. John of God (1495–1550)
Juana of the Cross,

Louise Lateau, Belgium (1850–83),
Blessed Lucy of Narni
Lukardis of Obermeyer (1276–1309)
St. Lydwine of Schiedam, Holland, (1380–1433)
Lutgarde,

Blessed Margaret Mary Alacoque, France (1647–90)
Margaret of Cortona
Margaret of the Blessed Sacrament
Maria Lopez of Jesus
Maria of the Incantation
Maria Dominica Lazzari (1815–48)
Marie-Julie Jahenny (1850–1941)
St. Marie
Marie Rose Ferron of North America (1902–36)
Marie de Moerl (1812–68)
Marthe Robbin (1902–81)
Mary Anne of Jesus
Mary Ellen Lukas of Hazelton, Pennsylvania (1954–Present)
St. Mary Frances of the Five Wounds (1715–91)
St. Mary Faustina Kowalska of Poland (1905–38)
Mary Magdalene de'Pazzi
Mary of Jesus Crucified
Matthew Carreri
Natuzza Evolo of Paravati, Italy (1924–2009)
Blessed Osanna of Mantua (1449–1505)
Padre Pio (1887–1962)
Rita of Cassia
Rita of Lima
St. Rose of Lima, Peru (1586–1617)
Stephana de Quinizanis
St. Teresa of Avila, Spain (1515–82)
Franciscan Tertiary (1557–1620)
Therese Neumann of Konnersreuth, Bavaria (1898–1962)
St. Veronica Giuliani (1660–1727)

ENDNOTES

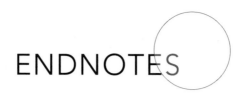

Introduction

1. Francois Rabelais, *Gargantua and Pantagruel, Book II*, trans. Sir Thomas Urquhart and Peter Anthony–Motteux (Hazelton, PA: Pennsylvania State University, Electronic Classics Series, 2006): 48.
2. F. J. Woodard, "A Phenomenological Study of Spontaneous Spiritual and Paranormal Experiencing in a 21st Century Sample of Normal People," *Psychological Reports* 110 (2012): 73–132.
3. F. J. Woodard, "Hypnosis and Phenomenological-Perceptual Psychology," *Journal of Clinical Psychology* 52, no. 2 (1996): 209–18. "Perceptually Oriented Hypnosis," *Psychological Reports* 92 (2003): 515–28. "Phenomenological Contributions to Understanding Hypnosis: Review of the Literature," *Psychological Reports* 93 (2003): 829–47. "An Argument for a Qualitative Research Approach to Hypnotic Experiencing and Perceptually Oriented Hypnosis," *Psychological Reports* 94 (2004): 955–66. "Response to Lynn, et al.'s Evaluation of 'Woodard's Theory of Perceptually Oriented Hypnosis,'" *Psychological Reports* 94 (2004): 431–36. "A Phenomenological and Perceptual Research Methodology for Understanding Hypnotic Experiencing," *Psychological Reports* 95 (2004): 887–904. "Perceptually Oriented Hypnosis: Cross-Cultural Perspectives," *Psychological Reports* 97 (2005): 141–57. "A Preliminary Phenomenological Study of Hypnotizing and Being Hypnotized," *Psychological Reports* 97 (2005): 423–66. "A Phenomenological Study of Spontaneous Spiritual and Paranormal Experiencing in a 21st Century Sample of Normal People," *Psychological Reports* 110 (2012): 73–132. "Perceptually Oriented Hypnosis: Removing a Socially Learned Pathology and Developing Adequacy: The Case of Invisible Girl," *Psychological Reports* 115 (2014): 545–64.
4. F. J. Woodard, "Family Tree Follies," *Nashua Telegraph* (2003, March 11): 18–19.
5. F. J. Woodard, *Searching for the Ancestors and Discovering the Descendants of Revolutionary War Captain Amos Woodard, a Great Grandson of Alfred the Great, Charlemagne, William the Conqueror, the Merovingian Kings and the House of Judah* (Milford, NH: Author, 2015).
6. F. J. Woodard, *Searching for the Ancestors and Discovering the Descendants of the Merovingian Kings, Chief Madockawando, Germain Lefebvre, Francois Chagnon, and My Grandmother Susan* Lefebvre (Milford, NH: Author, 2014).
7. L. Buscaglia, *Love* (New York, NY: Fawcett Crest, 1972), 10–11.

Chapter 1

8. C. Woodard, *A Doctor Heals by Faith* (London, England: William Clowes and Sons, 1953), 159.
9. F. J. Woodard, *A Phenomenological Inquiry of the Psychologist during the Hypnotic Experience* (Dissertation, California School of Professional Psychology, Ann Arbor, MI: University of Michigan, 2001).
10. D. Harvey, *The Power to Heal* (Wellingborough, Northamptonshire, England: Aquarian Press, 1983), 148.
11. D. Snygg and A. W. Combs, *Individual Behavior: A New Frame of Reference for Psychology* (New York, NY: Harper & Row, 1949), 15.

12. D. Snygg and A. W. Combs, *Individual Behavior: A Perceptual Approach to Behavior*, rev. ed. (New York, NY: Harper & Row, 1959), 28–29.

13. D. Snygg, "The Need for a Phenomenological System of Psychology," *Psychological Review* 48 (1941): 414.

14. D. G. Richards, "A Study of the Correlations between Subjective Psychic Experiences and Dissociative Experiences," *Dissociation* 4, no. 3 (1991): 83–91.

15. J. F. Schumaker, *The Corruption of Reality: A Unified Theory of Religion, Hypnosis, and Psychopathology* (Amherst, NY: Prometheus Books, 1995).

16. E. Taylor, *William James on Exceptional Mental States* (New York, NY: Charles Scribner's Sons, 1983), 6.

17. A.W. Combs, A.C. Richards, and F. Richards, *Perceptual Psychology: A Humanistic Approach to the Study of Persons* (Lanham, MD: University Press of America, 1988).

18. A.W. Combs, A.C. Richards, and F. Richards, *Perceptual Psychology: A Humanistic Approach to the Study of Persons* (Lanham, MD: University Press of America, 1988).

19. A.W. Combs, "Phenomenological Concepts in Nondirective Therapy," *Journal of Consulting Psychology* XII, no. 4 (1948): 201.

20. A.W. Combs, A.C. Richards, and F. Richards, *Perceptual Psychology: A Humanistic Approach to the Study of Persons* (Lanham, MD: University Press of America, 1988).

Chapter 2

21. S. M. Jourard, *The Transparent Self* (New York, NY: D. Van Nostrand Company, 1971), 93.

22. F. J. Woodard, "A Phenomenological Study of Spontaneous Spiritual and Paranormal Experiences in a 21st Century Sample of Normal People," *Psychological Reports* 110 (2012): 73–132.

23. P. Tillich, *The Courage to Be* (New Haven, CT: Yale University Press, 1952), 59.

24. F. J. Woodard, *Searching for the Ancestors and Discovering the Descendants of the Merovingian Kings, Chief Madockawando, Germain Lefebvre, Francois Chagnon, and My Grandmother Susan Lefebvre* (Milford, NH: Author, 2014).

25. D. Snygg and A. W. Combs, *Individual Behavior: A New Frame of Reference for Psychology* (New York, NY: Harper & Row, 1949), 88.

26. I. Stevenson, *Children Who Remember Previous Lives* (Charlottesville, VA: The University Press of Virginia, 1987).

27. J. Fort, "Mind Control: The What and How of Conversion and Indoctrination ('Brainwashing')," In *Clinical Hypnosis in Medicine*, ed. H. J. Wain, 219–27 (Chicago: Yearbook Medical Publishers, 1980), 220.

28. K. E. Boulding, *The Image* (Ann Arbor, MI: University of Michigan Press, 1969), 141.

Chapter 3

29. O. Rank, *The Psychology and the Soul*, trans. William D. Turner (Philadelphia, PA: University of Pennsylvania Press, 1950), 87.

30. "Trance," Merriam-Webster Dictionary, http://www.merriam-webster.com/dictionary/trance.

31. J. Wyckoff, *Franz Anton Mesmer: Between God and Devil* (Englewood Cliffs, NJ: Prentice-Hall, 1975), 23.

32. M. W. Calkins, ed., *Berkeley Essay, Principles, Dialogues with Selections from Other Writings* (New York, NY: Charles Scribner's Sons, 1957), 33.

33. M. W. Calkins, ed., *Berkeley Essay, Principles, Dialogues with Selections from Other Writings* (New York, NY: Charles Scribner's Sons, 1957), 33.

34. L. Buscaglia, *Love* (New York, NY: Fawcett Crest, 1972), 169.
35. A. A. Sheikh and C. S. Jordan, "Clinical Uses of Mental Imagery," in *Imagery, Current Theory, Research and Application*, ed. A. A. Sheikh (New York, NY: John Wiley & Sons, 1983), 393.
36. A. Spraggett, "Toronto Test of Ted Serios' Paranormal Photographs," *Fate*, (1965)
37. A. Puharich, *Beyond Telepathy* (Garden City, NY: Doubleday & Co., Inc., 1962).
38. J. W. Woodard, *Intellectual Realism and Culture Change. A Preliminary Study of Reification* (Hanover, NH: The Sociological Press, 1935), 56, 58–59.
39. E. Taylor, *William James on Exceptional Mental States* (New York, NY: Charles Scribner's Sons, 1983).

Chapter 4

40. G. Vermes, *The Complete Dead Sea Scrolls in English* (London, England: Penguin Books, 2004), 103.
41. W. Penfield, *The Mystery of the Mind* (Princeton, NJ: Princeton University Press, 1975), 35.
42. A. W. Combs, A. C. Richards, and F. Richards, *Perceptual Psychology: A Humanistic Approach to the Study of Persons* (Lanham, MD: University Press of America, 1988), 57.
43. C. E. Moustakas, *Phenomenological Research Methods* (San Diego, CA: Sage Publications, 1994), 26.
44. L. Binswanger, "The Case of Ellen West," In *Existence: A New Dimension in Psychiatry and Psychology*, eds. R. May, E. Angle, H. F. Ellenberger (New York, NY: Basic Books, 1958), 327.
45. S. B. Kopp, *Guru: Metaphors from a Psychotherapist* (Palo Alto, CA: Science and Behavior Books, 1971), 12.
46. L. Buscaglia, *Love* (New York, NY: Fawcett Crest, 1972).

Chapter 5

47. F. Franck, *The Zen of Seeing* (New York, NY: Vintage Books, 1973), 112.
48. M. Baigent, R. Leigh, and H. Lincoln, *The Messianic Legacy* (New York, NY: Delta Trade, 2004), 199.
49. A. W. Combs, A. C. Richards, and F. Richards, *Perceptual Psychology: A Humanistic Approach to the Study of Persons* (New York, NY: Harper & Row, 1976).
50. J. Haley, *Conversations with Milton H. Erickson, M.D., Volume I: Changing Individuals* (New York, NY: Triangle Press, 1985), 121.

Chapter 6

51. J. Fort, "Mind Control: The What and How of Conversion and Indoctrination ('Brainwashing')," in *Clinical Hypnosis in Medicine*, ed. H. J. Wain, 219–27 (Chicago, IL: Yearbook Medical Publishers, 1980), 226.
52. L. F. Cooper and M. H. Erickson, *The Clinical and Therapeutic Applications of Time Distortion* (Baltimore, MD: Williams & Wilkins, 1954), 44.
53. F. J. Woodard, "Hypnosis and Phenomenological-Perceptual Psychology," *Journal of Clinical Psychology* 52, no. 2 (1996): 213.
54. J. P. Zubek, *Sensory Deprivation: Fifteen Years of Research* (New York, NY: Appelton-Century-Crofts, 1969).
55. G. Orwell, *Nineteen Eighty-Four* (New York, NY: New American Library, 1964).
56. American Psychiatric Association, *Diagnostic and Statistical Manual of Mental Disorders*, 4th ed. (Washington, DC: Author, 1994), 768.

57. R. S. Broughton, *Parapsychology: The Controversial Science* (New York, NY: Ballantine Books, 1991), 35.

58. M. Baigent, *Exposing the Greatest Cover Up in History: The Jesus Papers* (New York, NY: Harper Collins, 2006), 204.

59. S. Krippner, "Conflicting Perspectives on Shamans and Shamanism: Points and Counterpoints," *American Psychologist* 57, no. 11 (2002): 962–77.

60. A. E. Bergin, "Psychotherapy and Religious Values," *Journal of Consulting and Clinical Psychology* 48, no. 1 (1980): 98.

61. A. W. Combs, "Phenomenological Concepts in Nondirective Therapy," *Journal of Consulting Psychology* 12, no. 4 (1948): 197–208.

62. D. Snygg and A. W. Combs, *Individual Behavior: A New Frame of Reference for Psychology* (New York, NY: Harper & Row, 1949), 165.

63. P. W. Sheehan and K. M. McConkey, *Hypnosis and Experience: The Exploration of Phenomena and Process* (Hillsdale, NJ: Lawrence Erlbaum, 1982).

64. W. Kroger, "Introduction and Supplemental Reports on Hypnoanesthesia," In *Hypnosis in Medicine and Surgery*, ed. J. Esdaile (New York, NY: The Julian Press, 1850/1957).

65. T. Elliotson, *Numerous Cases of Surgical Operations without Pain in the Mesmeric State* (Philadelphia, PA: Lea & Blanchard, 1843).

66. W. Kroger, "Introduction and Supplemental Reports on Hypnoanesthesia," In *Hypnosis in Medicine and Surgery* ed. J. Esdaile (New York, NY: The Julian Press, 1850/1957).

67. D. Snygg and A. W. Combs, *Individual Behavior: A New Frame of Reference for Psychology* (New York, NY: Harper & Row, 1949), 56–57.

68. S. Fisher, "The Role of Expectancy in the Performance of Post-hypnotic Behavior," *Journal of Abnormal and Social Psychology*, 49 (1954): 503–7.

69. K. S. Bowers, *Hypnosis for the Seriously Curious* (New York, NY: W. W. Norton & Company, 1976), 17–18.

70. A. W. Combs, A. C. Richards, and F. Richards, *Perceptual Psychology: A Humanistic Approach to the Study of Persons* (New York, NY: Harper & Row, 1976), 105.

71. H. J. Eysenck, *Sense and Nonsense in Psychology* (Harmondsworth, England: Penguin Books, 1964), 43–44.

72. F. J. Woodard, "Hypnosis and Phenomenological-Perceptual Psychology," *Journal of Clinical Psychology*, 52, no. 2 (1996): 212.

Chapter 7

73. J. Haley, *Conversations with Milton H. Erickson, M.D.,* Volume I: *Changing Individuals* (New York, NY: Triangle Press, 1985), 269.

74. D. Snygg and A. W. Combs, *Individual Behavior: A New Frame of Reference for Psychology* (New York, NY: Harper & Row, 1949).

75. A. H. Maslow, *Religions, Values, and Peak-Experiences* (New York, NY: Penguin Books, 1994), 75.

76. L. Buscaglia, *Love* (New York, NY: Fawcett Crest, 1972), 80.

Chapter 8

77. J. W. Woodard, *Intellectual Realism and Culture Change: A Preliminary Study of Reification* (Hanover, NH: The Sociological Press, 1935), 35.

78. L. F. Cooper and M. H. Erickson, *The Clinical and Therapeutic Applications of Time Distortion* (Baltimore, MD: Williams & Wilkins, 1954), 86.

79. J. S. Bruner and C. G. Goodman, "Value and Need as Organizing Factors of Perception," *Journal of Abnormal and Social Psychology* 42 (1947): 33–44.
80. D. Snygg, "The Need for a Phenomenological System of Psychology," *Psychological Review* 48 (1941): 414.
81. J. W. Woodard, "A New Classification of Culture and a Restatement of the Culture Lag Theory," *American Sociological Review* 1 (1936): 99.
82. W. Sargant, *Battle for the Mind: A Physiology of Conversion and Brain Washing* (Cambridge, MA: Malor Books, 1997).
83. S. J. Gould, "Advertising and Hypnotic Suggestion: The Construct of Advertising Suggestion," In *Human Suggestibility: Advances in Theory, Research, and Application*, ed. J. F. Schumaker (New York, NY: Routledge, 1991), 346.
84. C. Merrill, "You Are Getting Sleepy," *American Demographics* 21, no. 12 (December, 1999): 12–14.
85. E. Fromm, *To Have or To Be?* (New York, NY: Harper, 1975), 110.
86. W. W. Cook, *Practical Lessons in Hypnotism* (New York, NY: Willey Book Company, 1927), 201.
87. C. Sextus, *Hypnotism* (Hollywood, CA: Wilshire Book Company, 1957), 65.
88. R. C. Sprinthall, *Basic Statistical Analysis*, 4th ed. (Needham Heights, MA: Allyn and Bacon, 1994).
89. J. Monahan and R. W. Novaco, "Corporate Violence: A Psychological Analysis," in *New Directions in Psychological Research*, ed. P. Lipsitt and B. Sales. (New York, NY: Van Nostrand, 1980).
90. W. Sargant, *Battle for the Mind: A Physiology of Conversion and Brain Washing* (Cambridge, MA: Malor Books, 1997), 79–80.
91. W. B. Key, *The Clam Plate Orgy* (Englewood Cliffs, NJ: Prentice-Hall, 1980).
92. R. C. Sprinthall, personal communication, April 28, 1997.
93. G. H. Estabrooks, *Hypnotism* (New York, NY: E. P. Dutton & Co., 1957), 42.
94. S. J. Gould, "Advertising and Hypnotic Suggestion: The Construct of Advertising Suggestion," In *Human Suggestibility: Advances in Theory, Research, and Application*, ed. J. F. Schumaker (New York, NY: Routledge, 1991).
95. S. L. Hwang, "'Smoxploitation' Films Signal That Smoking Is Becoming a Fetish among Many," *Wall Street Journal* 1 (1996): A4.
96. R. L. Spitzer, M. Gibbon, A. E. Skodol, J. B. W. Williams, and M. B. First, eds., *DSM-IV Casebook* (Washington, DC: American Psychiatric Press, 1994).
97. R. L. Spitzer, M. Gibbon, A. E. Skodol, J. B. W. Williams, and M. B. First, eds., *DSM-IV Casebook* (Washington, DC: American Psychiatric Press, 1994), 80.

Chapter 9

98. L. J. Phillips and J.W. Osborne, "Cancer Patients' Experiences of Forgiveness Therapy," *Canadian Journal of Counseling* 23, no. 3 (1989): 238.
99. D. Radin, *The Conscious Universe* (San Francisco, CA: Harper Edge Publications, 1997), 112–13.
100. G. Livneh, "An Ostensible Precognition of the Arab Surprise Attack on the Day of Atonement, 1973," *Journal of Parapsychology* 53 (1986): 383–86.
101. F. J. Woodard, "A Phenomenological Study of Spontaneous Spiritual and Paranormal Experiences in a 21st Century Sample of Normal People," *Psychological Reports* 110 (2012): 73–132.
102. C. B. Ruffin, *Padre Pio: The True Story* (Huntington, IN: Our Sunday Visitor, 1991).
103. R. Wain, "Pain Control through the Use of Hypnosis," *American Journal of Clinical Hypnosis* 23, no. 1 (1980): 41–46.

104. *King James Version of the Holy Bible* (New York, NY: Thomas Nelson Publishers, 1976), 1690–91.

105. T. Okley, ed., *The Little Flowers of St. Francis* (London, England: J. M. Dent and Sons, 1910), 160.

106. O. D. Ratnoff, "Stigmata: Where Mind and Body Meet," *Medical Times* 97 (1969): 150–63.

107. A. Docker, "Wholism and Health—The Mind/Body Relationship," *Access, The Journal of ABH & the ABNLP and TLTA* (Spring, 2005): 16.

108. P. Tillich, *The Courage to Be* (New Haven, CT: Yale University Press, 1952), 49–50.

109. E. Taylor, *William James on Exceptional Mental States* (New York, NY: Charles Scribner's Sons, 1983), 129.

110. *King James Version of the Holy Bible* (New York, NY: Thomas Nelson Publishers, 1976), 1414.

111. J. B. Tucker, *Life before Life: A Scientific Investigation of Children's Memories of Previous Lives* (New York, NY: St. Martin's Press, 2005).

112. L. F. Early and J. E. Lifschutz, "A Case of Stigmata," *Archives of General Psychiatry* 30 (1974): 197–200.

113. M. Freze, *They Bore the Wounds of Christ* (Huntington, IN: Our Sunday Visitor, 1989).

114. K. L. Woodward, *Making Saints: How the Catholic Church Determines Who Becomes a Saint, Who Doesn't, and Why* (New York, NY: Simon & Schuster, 1990).

115. R. L. Moody, "Bodily Changes in Abreaction," *Lancet 248* (1946): 934–35.

116. R. L. Moody, "Bodily Changes in Abreaction," *Lancet 248* (1946): 934–35.

117. R. Menzies, "Further Studies of Conditioned Vasomotor Responses in Human Subjects," *Journal of Experimental Psychology* 29 (1941): 457.

118. P. Siwek, *The Riddle of Konnersreuth* (Dublin, Ireland: Browne and Nolan, 1954).

119. R. Biot, *The Riddle of the Stigmata* (London, England: Burns Oates, 1962).

120. F. A. Whitlock and J.V. Hynes, "Religious Stigmatization: An Historical and Psychophysiological Enquiry," *Psychological Medicine* 8 (1978): 185–202.

121. J. E. Lifschutz, "Hysterical Stigmatization," *American Journal of Psychiatry* 114 (1957): 527–31.

122. L. F. Early and J. E. Lifschutz, "A Case of Stigmata," *Archives of General Psychiatry* 30 (1974): 197–200.

123. C. Hull, *Hypnosis and Suggestibility: An Experimental Approach* (New York, NY: Appleton-Century Crofts, 1933).

124. W. Needles, "Stigmata Occurring in the Course of Psychoanalysis," *Psychoanalytic Quarterly* 12 (1943): 23–39.

125. M. Ullman, "Herpes Simplex and Second Degree Burns Induced under Hypnosis," *American Journal of Psychiatry* 103 (1947), 828–30.

126. J. B. Tucker, *Life before Life: A Scientific Investigation of Children's Memories of Previous Lives* (New York, NY: St. Martin's Press, 2005).

127. C. J. Simpson, "The Stigmata: Pathology or Miracle?" *British Medical Journal* 289 (1984): 1746–48.

128. R. A. Lord, "A Note on Stigmata," *American Imago* 14 (1957): 299–301.

129. F. A. Whitlock and J. V. Hynes, "Religious Stigmatization: An Historical and Psychophysiological Enquiry," *Psychological Medicine* 8 (1978): 185–202.

130. R. A. Lord, "A Note on Stigmata," *American Imago* 14 (1957): 299–301.

131. O. D. Ratnoff, "Stigmata: Where Mind and Body Meet," *Medical Times* 97 (1969): 163.

132. R. Bach, *Illusions: The Adventure of a Reluctant Messiah* (New York, NY: Dell Publishing, 1979), 49.

133. D. B. Bradley and R. A. Bradley, *Psychic Phenomena: Revelations and Experiences* (West Nyack, NY: Parker, 1967/1971), 39.

134. A. H. Maslow, "Isomorphic Interrelationships Between Knower and Known," in *Sign, Image, Symbol*, ed. G. Kepes (New York, NY: Braziller, 1966), 134.

135. W. S. Kroger, *Clinical and Experimental Hypnosis* (Philadelphia, PA: J. B. Lippincott Company, 1977), 122.

136. R. Copelan, *How to Hypnotize Yourself and Others* (New York, NY: Harper & Row Publishers, 1981), 189.

137. W. J. Bryan, *Leave Something to God: The Religious Aspects of Hypnosis* (Winfield, IL: Relaxed Books, 1962).

138. I. C. Beveridge, *Hypnotherapy: Its Christian Aspects* (Columbus, GA: Brentwood Christian Press, 1992), 33.

139. *King James Version of the Holy Bible* (New York, NY: Thomas Nelson Publishers, 1976).

140. C. B. Ruffin, *Padre Pio: The True Story* (Huntington, IN: Our Sunday Visitor, 1991).

141. G. Egan, *The Skilled Helper: A Problem-Management Approach to Helping* (Pacific Grove, CA: Brookes/Cole Publishing, 1994), 15.

142. S. Keen, "Original Blessing, Not Original Sin," *Psychology Today* (June, 1989): 57.

143. J.C. Pearce, *The Crack in the Cosmic Egg* (New York, NY: Pocket Books, 1974), 106.

144. E. Taylor, *William James on Exceptional Mental States* (New York, NY: Charles Scribner's Sons, 1983), 125.

145. F. Franck, *The Zen of Seeing* (New York, NY: Vintage Books, 1973), 113.

Chapter 10

146. A. H. Maslow, *Religions, Values, and Peak-Experiences* (New York, NY: Penguin Books, 1994), 32.

147. W. G. Roll, *The Poltergeist* (Metuchen, NJ: Scarecrow Press, 1972), 12.

148. W. G. Roll, *The Poltergeist* (Metuchen, NJ: Scarecrow Press, 1972), 194.

149. A. Greeley, "Mysticism Goes Mainstream" *American Health* 6, no. 1 (1987): 41–49.

150. E. Haraldsson, A. Gudmundsdottir, A. Ragnarsson, J. Loftsson, and S. Jonsson, "National Survey of Psychical Experiences and Attitudes towards The Paranormal In Iceland," In *Research in Parapsychology 1976*, ed. J. D. Morris, W. G. Roll, and R. L. Morris (Metuchen, NJ: Scarecrow Press, 1977).

151. C. Sextus, *Hypnotism* (Hollywood, CA: Wilshire Book Company, 1957), 176.

152. E. Gabor, *Home at the Tree of Life: An Introduction to Subconscious, Ethereal Science* (Middletown, DE: Author, 2013)

153. J. E. Kennedy, H. Kanthamani, and J. Palmer, "Psychic and Spiritual Experiences, Health, Well Being and Meaning in Life," *Journal of Parapsychology* 58 (1994): 353–83.

154. M. H. Erickson, *The Collected Papers of Milton H. Erickson. Vol. IV: Innovative Hypnotherapy*, ed. E. L. Rossi (New York, NY: Irvington, 1989), xviii.

155. R.A. Moody, *Life after Life* (New York, NY: Bantam Books, 1975), 65.

156. I. Stevenson, *Children Who Remember Previous Lives* (Charlottesville, VA: The University Press of Virginia, 1987), 230.

157. F. J. Woodard "A Phenomenological Study of Spontaneous Spiritual and Paranormal Experiencing in a 21st Century Sample of Normal People," *Psychological Reports* 110 (2012): 73–132.

158. E. Servadio, *Psychology Today* (New York, NY: Garrett & Helix, 1965).

159. B. Schwartz, *Psychic Dynamics* (New York, NY: Pageant Press, 1965).

160. J. Ehrenwald, *New Dimensions of Deep Analysis* (London, England: George Allen & Unwin, 1954).

161. J. Eisenbud, *Psi and Psychoanalysis* (New York, NY: Grune & Stratto, 1970).

162. J. Eisenbud, *Parapsychology and the Unconscious* (Berkeley, CA: North Atlantic, 1992).

163. J. W. Woodard, *Intellectual Realism and Culture Change. A Preliminary Study of Reification* (Hanover, NH: The Sociological Press, 1935), 66.

164. J. D. Frank, *Persuasion and Healing: A Comparative Study of Psychotherapy* (New York, NY: Schocken Books, 1974), 335.

165. W. W. Cook, *Practical Lessons in Hypnotism* (New York, NY: Willey Book Company, 1927), 233.

166. C. Sextus, *Hypnotism* (Hollywood, CA: Wilshire Book Company, 1957).

167. P. Wanis, *Look into My Eyes* (Boca Raton, FL: American Media Mini Mags, 2002).

168. W. James, *The Varieties of Religious Experience* (New York, NY: Mentor Books, 1958), 98.

169. J. H. Slate, *Psychic Vampires: Protection from Energy Predators and Parasites* (St. Paul, MN: Llewellyn Publications, 2002). 223.

170. D. B. Bradley and R. A. Bradley, *Psychic Phenomena: Revelations and Experiences* (West Nyack, NY: Parker Publishing, 1967/1971), 61.

171. M. Newton, *Journey of Souls, Case Studies of Life between Lives* (St. Paul, Minnesota: Llewellyn Publications, 1995).

172. S. Modi, *Memories of God and Creation* (Charlottesville, VA: Hampton Books, 2000).

173. I. Stevenson, "Cryptomnesia and Parapsychology," *Journal of the Society of Psychical Research* 52 (1983): 1–30.

174. D. Sutphen, *Past Lives, Future Loves* (New York: Pocket Books, 1978).

175. R.J. Woolger, *Other Lives, Other Selves* (New York, NY: Bantam Books, 1988).

176. L. Tarazi, "An Unusual Case of Hypnotic Regression with Some Unexplained Contents," *Journal of American Society for Psychical Research* 84, no. 4 (1990): 328.

177. M. Bernstein, *The Search for Bridey Murphy* (Garden City, NY: Doubleday, 1956).

178. M. V. Kline, ed. *A Scientific Report on "The Search for Bridey Murphy"* (New York, NY: Julian, 1956).

179. M. A. Gravitz, "The Search for Bridey Murphy: Implications for Modern Hypnosis," *American Journal of Clinical Hypnosis* 45, no. 1 (2002): 3–10.

180. C. J. Ducasse, "How the Case of the Search for Bridey Murphy Stands Today," *Journal of American Society of Psychical Research* 54 (1960): 3–22.

181. C. J. Ducasse, "How the Case of the Search for Bridey Murphy Stands Today," *Journal of American Society of Psychical Research* 54 (1960): 3–22.

Chapter 11

182. P. Tillich, *The Courage to Be* (New Haven, CT: Yale University Press, 1952), 115.

183. D. Snygg and A. W. Combs, *Individual Behavior: A New Frame of Reference for Psychology* (New York, NY: Harper & Row, 1949), 247.

184. D. Snygg and A. W. Combs, *Individual Behavior: A New Frame of Reference for Psychology* (New York, NY: Harper & Row, 1949), 128.

185. F. J. Woodard, "Perceptually Oriented Hypnosis: Removing a Socially Learned Pathology and Developing Adequacy: The Case of Invisible Girl," *Psychological Reports* 115 (2014): 545–64.

186. D. Snygg and A. W. Combs, *Individual Behavior: A New Frame of Reference for Psychology* (New York, NY: Harper & Row, 1949).

BIBLIOGRAPHY

American Psychiatric Association. *Diagnostic and Statistical Manual of Mental Disorders*. 4th edition. Washington, DC: Author, 1994.

Bach, R. *Illusions: The Adventure of a Reluctant Messiah*. New York, NY: Dell Publishing, 1977.

Baigent, M. *Exposing the Greatest Cover Up in History: The Jesus Papers*. New York, NY: Harper Collins, 2007.

Baigent, M., R. Leigh, and H. Lincoln. *The Messianic Legacy*. New York, NY: Delta Trade, 2004.

Bergin, A. E. 1980. "Psychotherapy and Religious Values." *Journal of Consulting and Clinical Psychology* 48 (1): 95–105.

Bernstein, M. *The Search for Bridey Murphy*. Garden City, NY: Doubleday, 1956.

Beveridge, I. C. *Hypnotherapy: Its Christian Aspects*. Columbus, GA: Brentwood Christian Press, 1992.

Binswanger, L. "The Case of Ellen West." In *Existence: A New Dimension in Psychiatry and Psychology*, ed. R. May, E. Angle, and H. F. Ellenberger, 237–364. New York, NY: Basic Books, 1958.

Biot, R. *The Riddle of the Stigmata*. London, England: Burns Oates, 1962.

Borenzweig, H. "Touching in Clinical Social Work." *Social Casework* 64 (1983): 238–42.

Boulding, K. E. *The Image*. Ann Arbor, MI: University of Michigan Press, 1969.

Bowers, K. S. *Hypnosis for the Seriously Curious*. New York, NY: W. W. Norton & Company, 1976.

Bradley, D. B., and R. A. Bradley. *Psychic Phenomena: Revelations and Experiences*. West Nyack, NY: Parker Publishing, 1967/1971.

Breuer, J., and S. Freud. *Studies in Hysteria*. London, England: Hogarth Press, 1955.

Broughton, R. S. *Parapsychology: The Controversial Science*. New York, NY: Ballantine Books, 1991.

Bruner, J. S. *A Study in Thinking*. New York, NY: Science Editions, 1962.

Bruner, J. S., and C. G. Goodman. "Value and Need as Organizing Factors of Perception." *Journal of Abnormal and Social Psychology* 42 (1947): 33–44.

Bryan, W. J. *Leave Something to God: The Religious Aspects of Hypnosis*. Winfield, IL: Relaxed Books, 1962.

Buscaglia, L. *Love*. New York, NY: Fawcett Crest, 1972.

Calkins, M. W., ed. *Berkeley Essay, Principles, Dialogues with Selections from Other Writings*. New York, NY: Charles Scribner's Sons, 1957.

Carty, C. M. *The Stigmata and Modern Science*. Rockford, IL: Tan Books and Publishers, 1974.

Combs, A. W. "Phenomenological Concepts in Nondirective Therapy." *Journal of Consulting Psychology* 12 (4; 1948): 197–208.

Combs, A. W., A. C. Richards, and F. Richards. *Perceptual Psychology: A Humanistic Approach to the Study of Persons*. New York, NY: Harper & Row, 1976.

Cook, W. W. *Practical Lessons in Hypnotism*. New York, NY: Willey Book Company, 1927.

Cooper, L. F., and M. H. Erickson. *The Clinical and Therapeutic Applications of Time Distortion*. Baltimore, MD: Williams & Wilkins, 1954.

Copelan, R. *How to Hypnotize Yourself and Others*. New York, NY: Harper & Row, 1981.

Coue, E. *Better and Better Every Day*. London, England: Unwin Books, 1961.

Docker, A. "Holism and Health—The Mind/Body Relationship." *Access, The Journal of ABH & the ABNLP and TLTA* (Spring 2005).

Ducasse, C. J. "How the Case of the Search for Bridey Murphy Stands Today." *Journal of American Society of Psychical Research* 54 (1960): 3–22.

Early, L. F., and J. E. Lifschutz. "A Case of Stigmata." *Archives of General Psychiatry* 30 (1974): 197–200.

Egan, G. *The Skilled Helper: A Problem-Management Approach to Helping.* Pacific Grove, CA: Brookes/Cole Publishing, 1994.

Ehrenwald, J. *New Dimensions of Deep Analysis.* London, England: George Allen & Unwin, 1954.

Eisenbud, J. *Psi and Psychoanalysis.* New York, NY: Grune & Stratton, 1970.

Eisenbud, J. *Parapsychology and the Unconscious.* Berkeley, CA: North Atlantic Books, 1992.

Elliotson, T. *Numerous Cases of Surgical Operations Without Pain in the Mesmeric State.* Philadelphia, PA: Lea & Blanchard, 1843.

Erickson, M. *Advanced Techniques of Hypnosis and Therapy.* Edited by J. Haley. New York, NY: Grune & Stratton, 1967.

Erickson, M. H. *The Collected Papers of Milton H. Erickson. Vol. IV: Innovative Hypnotherapy.* Edited by E. L. Rossi. New York, NY: Irvington, 1989.

Estabrooks, G. H. *Hypnotism.* New York, NY: E. P. Dutton & Co., 1957.

Eysenck, H. J. *Sense and Nonsense in Psychology.* Harmondsworth, England: Penguin Books, 1964.

Fischer, C. "Individualized Assessment and Phenomenological Psychology." *Journal of Personality Assessment* 43 (2; 1979): 115–21.

Fisher, S. "The Role of Expectancy in the Performance of Post-hypnotic Behavior." *Journal of Abnormal and Social Psychology* 49 (1954): 503–7.

Fort, J. "Mind Control: The What and How of Conversion and Indoctrination ('Brainwashing')." In *Clinical Hypnosis in Medicine,* edited by H. J. Wain, 219–27. Chicago, IL: Yearbook Medical Publishers, 1980.

Franck, F. *The Zen of Seeing.* New York, NY: Vintage Books, 1973.

Frank, J. D. *Persuasion and Healing: A Comparative Study of Psychotherapy.* New York, NY: Schocken Books, 1974.

Freze, M. *They Bore the Wounds of Christ.* Huntington, IN: Our Sunday Visitor, 1989.

Fromm, E. *To Have or To Be?* New York, NY: Harper, 1975.

Gabor, E. *Home at the Tree of Life: An Introduction to Subconscious, Ethereal Science.* Middletown, DE: Author, 2013.

Goleman, D. *Emotional Intelligence.* New York, NY: Bantam Books, 1995.

Gould, S. J. "Advertising and Hypnotic Suggestion: The Construct of Advertising Suggestion." In *Human Suggestibility: Advances in Theory, Research, and Application,* edited by J. F. Schumaker, 341–58. New York, NY: Routledge, 1991.

Gravitz, M. A. "The Search for Bridey Murphy: Implications for Modern Hypnosis." *American Journal of Clinical Hypnosis* 45 (1; 2002): 3–10.

Greeley, A. "Mysticism Goes Mainstream." *American Health* 6 (1; 1987): 41–49.

Haley, J. *Conversations with Milton H. Erickson, M.D. Vol. I: Changing Individuals.* New York, NY: Triangle Press, 1985.

Haraldsson, E., A. Gudmundsdottir, A. Ragnarsson, J. Loftsson, and S. Jonsson. "National Survey of Psychic Experiences and Attitudes towards the Paranormal in Iceland." In *Research in Parapsychology 1976,* edited by J. D. Morris, W. G. Roll, and R. L. Morris. Metuchen, NJ: Scarecrow Press, 1977.

Harrison, T. *Stigmata: A Medieval Mystery in a Modern Age.* New York, NY: St. Martin's Press, 1994.

Harvey, D. *The Power to Heal.* Wellingborough, Northamptonshire, England: Aquarian Press, 1983.

Hull, C. *Hypnosis and Suggestibility: An Experimental Approach.* New York, NY: Appleton-Century Crofts, 1933.

Hwang, S. L. "'Smoxploitation' Films Signal That Smoking Is Becoming a Fetish among Many." *Wall Street Journal* 1 (1996): A4.

James, W. *The Varieties of Religious Experience.* New York, NY: Mentor Books, 1958.

Jourard, S. M. *The Transparent Self.* New York, NY: D. Van Nostrand Company, 1971.

Keen, S. "Original Blessing, Not Original Sin." *Psychology Today*, June (1989): 54–58.

Kennedy, J. E., H. Kanthamani, and J. Palmer. 1994. "Psychic and Spiritual Experiences, Health, Well Being and Meaning in Life." *Journal of Parapsychology* 58: 353–83.

Key, W. B. *The Clam Plate Orgy*. Englewood Cliffs, NJ: Prentice-Hall, 1980.

King James Version of the Holy Bible. New York, NY: Thomas Nelson Publishers. 1976.

Kline, M. V., ed. *A Scientific Report on "The Search for Bridey Murphy."* New York, NY: Julian, 1956.

Kopp, S. B. *Guru: Metaphors from a Psychotherapist*. Palo Alto, CA: Science and Behavior Books, 1971.

Krippner, S. "Conflicting Perspectives on Shamans and Shamanism: Points and Counterpoints." *American Psychologist* 57 (11; 2002): 962–77.

Kroger, W. S. "Introduction and Supplemental Reports on Hypnoanesthesia." In *Hypnosis in Medicine and Surgery*, edited by J. Esdaile. New York, NY: The Julian Press, 1850/1957.

Kroger, W. S. *Clinical and Experimental Hypnosis*. Philadelphia, PA: J. B. Lippincott Company, 1977.

Lankton, S. *Practical Magic*. Cupertino, CA: Meta, 1980.

Lefkowitz, E. S., M. M. Gillen, C. L. Shearer, and T. L. Boone. "Religiosity, Sexual Behaviors, and Sexual Attitudes During Emerging Adulthood." *Journal of Sex Research* 41 (2004): 150–59.

Lifschutz, J. E. "Hysterical Stigmatization." *American Journal of Psychiatry* 114 (1954): 527–31.

Livneh, G. "An Ostensible Precognition of the Arab Surprise Attack on the Day of Atonement, 1973." *Journal of Parapsychology* 53 (1986): 383–86.

Lord, R. A. "A Note on Stigmata." *American Imago* 14 (1957): 299–301.

Maslow, A. H. "Isomorphic Interrelationships between Knower and Known." In *Sign, Image, Symbol*, edited by G. Kepes. New York, NY: Braziller, 1966.

Maslow, A. H. *Religions, Values, and Peak-Experiences*. New York, NY: Penguin Books, 1994.

Menzies, R. "Further Studies of Conditioned Vasomotor Responses in Human Subjects." *Journal of Experimental Psychology* 29 (1941): 457.

Merriam-Webster's Collegiate Dictionary, 11th edition. Springfield, MA: Merriam-Webster, 2015. http://www.merriam-webster.com/dictionary.

Merrill, C. "You Are Getting Sleepy." *American Demographics* 21 (12; 1999): 12–14.

Miller, G. E., and S. Cohen. "Psychological Interventions and the Immune System: A Meta-Analytic Review and Critique." *Health Psychology* 20 (1; 2001): 47–63.

Modi, S. *Memories of God and Creation*. Charlottesville, VA: Hampton Books, 2000.

Monahan, J., and R. W. Novaco. "Corporate Violence: A Psychological Analysis." In, *New Directions in Psychological Research*, edited by P. Lipsitt and B. Sales, 3–25. New York, NY: Van Nostrand, 1980.

Moody, R. L. "Bodily Changes in Abreaction." *Lancet* 248 (1946): 934–35.

Moody, R. A. *Life after Life*. New York, NY: Bantam Books, 1975.

Moustakas, C. E. *Phenomenological Research Methods*. San Diego, CA: Sage Publications, 1994.

Needles, W. "Stigmata Occurring in the Course of Psychoanalysis." *Psychoanalytic Quarterly* 12 (1943): 23–39.

Newton, M. *Journey of Souls, Case Studies of Life between Lives*. St. Paul, MN: Llewellyn Publications, 1995.

Okley, T., ed. *The Little Flowers of St. Francis*. London, England: J. M. Dent and Sons, 1910.

Orwell, G. *Nineteen Eighty-Four*. New York, NY: New American Library, 1964.

Pearce, J. C. *The Crack in the Cosmic Egg*. New York, NY: Pocket Books, 1974.

Penfield, W. *The Mystery of the Mind*. Princeton, NJ: Princeton University Press, 1975.

Puharich, A. *Beyond Telepathy*. Garden City, NY: Doubleday & Co., 1962.

Rabelais, F., c. 1494–1553. *Gargantua and Pantagruel Book II*. Translated by Sir Thomas Urquhart and Peter Anthony Motteux. Hazelton, PA: Pennsylvania State University, Electronic Classics Series, 2006.

Radin, D. *The Conscious Universe*. San Francisco, CA: Harper Edge Publications, 1997.

Rank, O. *The Psychology and the Soul*. Translated by William D. Turner. Philadelphia, PA: University of Pennsylvania Press, 1950.

Ratnoff, O. D. "Stigmata: Where Mind and Body Meet." *Medical Times* 97 (1969): 150–63.

Richards, A. C. "Humanistic Perspectives on Adequate and Artifactual Research." *Interpersonal Development* 1 (1970): 77–86.

Richards, D. G. "A Study of the Correlations between Subjective Psychic Experiences and Dissociative Experiences." *Dissociation* 4 (3; 1991): 83–91.

Roll, W. G. *The Poltergeist*. Metuchen, NJ: Scarecrow Press, 1972.

Ruffin, C. B. *Padre Pio: The True Story*. Huntington, IN: Our Sunday Visitor, 1991.

Sargant, W. *Battle for the Mind: A Physiology of Conversion and Brainwashing*. Cambridge, MA: Malor Books, 1997.

Schumaker, J. F. *The Corruption of Reality: A Unified Theory of Religion, Hypnosis, and Psychopathology*. Amherst, NY: Prometheus Books, 1995.

Schumaker, J. F., ed. *Human Suggestibility: Advances in Theory, Research and Application*. New York, NY: Routledge, 1991.

Schwartz, B. *Psychic Dynamics*. New York, NY: Pageant Press, 1965.

Servadio, E. *Psychology Today*. New York, NY: Garrett & Helix, 1965.

Sextus, C. *Hypnotism*. Hollywood, CA: Wilshire Book Company, 1957.

Sheehan, P. W., and K. M. McConkey. *Hypnosis and Experience: The Exploration of Phenomena and Process*. Hillsdale, NJ: Lawrence Erlbaum, 1982.

Sheikh, A. A., and C. S. Jordan. "Clinical Uses of Mental Imagery." In *Imagery, Current Theory, Research and Application*, edited by A. A. Sheikh. New York, NY: John Wiley & Sons, 1983.

Simpson, C. J. "The Stigmata: Pathology or Miracle?" *British Medical Journal* 289 (1984): 1746–48.

Siwek, P. (1954). *The Riddle of Konnersreuth*. Dublin, Ireland: Browne and Nolan.

Slate, J. H. (2002). *Psychic Vampires: Protection from Energy Predators and Parasites*. St. Paul, MN: Llewellyn Publications.

Slovenko, R. (1995). "Dreams as Evidence." *Journal of Psychiatry & Law* 23 (1): 191–201.

Snygg, D. (1941). "The Need for a Phenomenological System of Psychology." *Psychological Review* 48: 404–24.

Snygg, D., and A. W. Combs. (1949). *Individual Behavior: A New Frame of Reference for Psychology*. New York, NY: Harper & Row.

Snygg, D., and A. W. Combs. *Individual Behavior: A Perceptual Approach to Behavior*. Rev. ed. New York, NY: Harper & Row, 1959.

Spitzer, R. L., M. Gibbon, A. E. Skodol, J. B. W. Williams, and M. B. First, eds. *DSM-IV Casebook*. Washington, DC: American Psychiatric Press, 1994.

Spraggett, A. "Toronto Test of Ted Serios' Paranormal Photographs." *Fate*, 1965.

Sprinthall, R. C. *Basic Statistical Analysis*. 4th edition. Needham Heights, MA: Allyn and Bacon, 1994.

Stevenson, I. *Children Who Remember Previous Lives*. Charlottesville, VA: The University Press of Virginia, 1987.

Stevenson, I. "Cryptomnesia and Parapsychology." *Journal of the Society of Psychical Research* 52 (1983): 1–30.

Sutphen, D. *Past Lives, Future Loves*. New York, NY: Pocket Books, 1978.

Tarazi, L. "An Unusual Case of Hypnotic Regression with Some Unexplained Contents." *Journal of American Society for Psychical Research* 84 (4; 1990): 309–44.

Taylor, E. *William James on Exceptional Mental States*. New York, NY: Charles Scribner's Sons, 1983.

Tillich, P. *The Courage To Be*. New Haven, CT: Yale University Press, 1952.

Tucker, J. B. *Life before Life: A Scientific Investigation of Children's Memories of Previous Lives.* New York, NY: St. Martin's Press, 2005.

Ullman, M. "Herpes Simplex and Second Degree Burns Induced under Hypnosis." *American Journal of Psychiatry* 103 (1947): 828–30.

Vermes, G. *The Complete Dead Sea Scrolls in English.* London, England: Penguin Books, 2004.

Wain, R. "Pain Control through the Use of Hypnosis." *American Journal of Clinical Hypnosis* 23 (1; 1980): 41–46.

Wanis, P. *Look into My Eyes.* Boca Raton, FL: American Media Mini Mags, 2002.

Whitlock, F. A., and J. V. Hynes. "Religious Stigmatization: An Historical and Psychophysiological Enquiry." *Psychological Medicine* 8 (1978): 185–202.

Woodard, C. *A Doctor Heals by Faith.* London, England: William Clowes and Sons, 1953.

Woodard, F. J. "An Argument for a Qualitative Research Approach to Hypnotic Experiencing and Perceptually Oriented Hypnosis." *Psychological Reports* 94 (2004): 955–66.

Woodard, F. J. "Family Tree Follies." *Nashua Telegraph*, March 11, 2003.

Woodard, F. J. "Hypnosis and Phenomenological-Perceptual Psychology." *Journal of Clinical Psychology* 52 (2; 1996): 209–18.

Woodard, F. J. "Perceptually Oriented Hypnosis." *Psychological Reports* 92 (2003): 515–28.

Woodard, F. J. "Perceptually Oriented Hypnosis: Cross-Cultural Perspectives." *Psychological Reports* 97 (2005): 141–57.

Woodard, F. J. "Perceptually Oriented Hypnosis: Removing a Socially Learned Pathology and Developing Adequacy: The Case of Invisible Girl." *Psychological Reports* 115 (2014): 545–64.

Woodard, F. J. "Phenomenological Contributions to Understanding Hypnosis: Review of the Literature." *Psychological Reports* 93 (2003): 829–47.

Woodard, F. J. *A Phenomenological Inquiry of the Psychologist during the Hypnotic Experience.* Dissertation, California School of Professional Psychology, Ann Arbor, MI: University of Michigan, 2001.

Woodard, F. J. "A Phenomenological and Perceptual Research Methodology for Understanding Hypnotic Experiencing." *Psychological Reports* 95 (2004): 877–904.

Woodard, F. J. "A Preliminary Phenomenological Study of Hypnotizing and Being Hypnotized." *Psychological Reports* 97 (2005): 423–66.

Woodard, F. J. "A Phenomenological Study of Spontaneous Spiritual and Paranormal Experiencing in a 21st Century Sample of Normal People." *Psychological Reports* 110 (2012): 73–132.

Woodard, F. J. "Response to Beshai's 'Quantitative and Qualitative Research in Hypnosis: Comment on Woodard,'" *Psychological Reports* 98 (2006): 908–10.

Woodard, F. J. "Response to Lynn et al.'s Evaluation of Woodard's Theory of Perceptually Oriented Hypnosis." *Psychological Reports* 94 (2004): 431–36.

Woodard, F. J. *Searching for the Ancestors and Discovering the Descendants of Revolutionary War Captain Amos Woodard, a Great Grandson of Charlamagne, William the Conquerer, or Merovingian Kings and House of Judah.* Milford, NH: Author, 2015.

Woodard, J. W. "A New Classification of Culture and a Restatement of the Culture Lag Theory." *American Sociological Review* 1 (1936): 89–102.

Woodard, J. W. "Critical Notes on the Nature of Sociology as a Science." *Social Forces* 11 (1; 1932): 28–43.

Woodard, J. W. *Intellectual Realism and Culture Change. A Preliminary Study of Reification.* Hanover, NH: The Sociological Press, 1935.

Woodward, K. L. *Making Saints: How the Catholic Church Determines Who Becomes a Saint, Who Doesn't, and Why.* New York, NY: Simon & Schuster, 1990.

Woolger, R. J. *Other Lives, Other Selves.* New York, NY: Bantam Books, 1988.

Wyckoff, J. Franz. *Anton Mesmer: Between God and Devil.* Englewood Cliffs, NJ: Prentice-Hall, 1975.

Zubek, J. P. *Sensory Deprivation: Fifteen Years of Research.* New York, NY: Appleton Century Crofts, 1969.

ABOUT THE AUTHOR

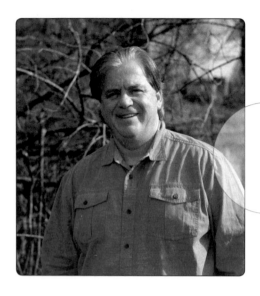

Dr. Fredrick Woodard received a Doctorate of Clinical Hypnotherapy from the American Institute of Hypnotherapy in 1992, a Doctorate of Philosophy in Clinical Psychology from the California School of Professional Psychology in 2002, and underwent intensive training at the Milton Erickson Institute in Arizona. He received the New England Paranormal Researcher of the Year award in 2012 from CeCe Productions. He is a registered and certified clinical hypnotherapist and has been a member of the American Board of Hypnotherapy, American Psychological Association, New Hampshire Psychological Association, the Society for Scientific Exploration, and APA—Psychological Hypnosis. Dr. Woodard was deployed for a month in Louisiana during the Katrina disaster in 2005. He is a direct great-grandchild of Chief Madockawando of the Abenaki Nation, Charlamagne, and the Merovingian Kings.